Let's Play Doctor

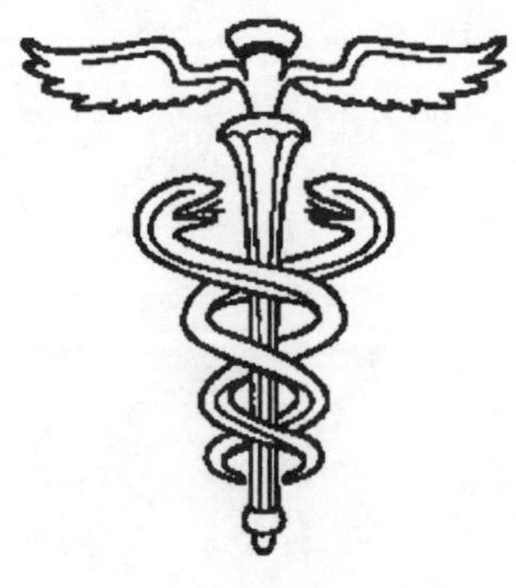

Let's Play Doctor

Joel D. Wallach, BS, DVM, ND
Ma Lan, MD, MS

The information in this book is intended to be medical instruction. It's purpose is to be educational and informative. It is assumed the user, as their own primary health care provider, will consult with or refer themselves to an N.D., D.C., or D.V.M. as they deem necessary.

Library of Congress Cataloging in Publications Data:

Wallach, J.D. and Lan, Ma
LET'S PLAY DOCTOR
Bibliography: p
Includes Index

1. Wholistic Health Care.
2. Self-Help Health Care.
3. Translations -prescriptions.
5. Eclectic Materia Medica.
6. Alternative Self-Help

LET'S PLAY DOCTOR
First Edition, 1989
Second Edition, 1991
Third Edition, 1997

Printed and published by:
Double Happiness Publishing Co., Bonita, CA

Acknowledgement

The extraordinary help and technical advice of Vince Marasigan, Linda Wick and the staff of the Double Happiness Publishing Company allowed us to have a joyous "home delivery." We also need to thank my 13 year-old son, Jeremiah C. Wallach for doing a significant amount of grunt work on the rough manuscripts.

"I am a realist, as long as the profit is in the treatment of symptoms rather than in the search for causes, that's where the medical profession will go for it's harvest."

— ARTHUR F. COCA, M.D.
The Pulse Test

Dedication

This book is dedicated to individual health freedom, freedom of choice in health care, the Constitution of the United States and to the separation of medicine and state as with church and state.

"The Constitution of this Republic should make special provisions for Medical Freedom as well as Religious Freedom. To restrict the art of healing to one class of men and deny equal privileges to others will constitute the Bastille of medical science. All such laws are unAmerican and despotic."

— **BENJAMIN RUSH, M.D.**
A signer of the Declaration of Independence and this nation's first Surgeon General

Table of Contents

Introduction Peter & Jacqueline Holliday xi

Foreword Lendon Smith, M.D. xiii

Preface Joel D. Wallach, B.S., D.V.M., N.D. xv

Chapter 1 Pre-Med 1

Chapter 2 Doctor Talk 11

Chapter 3 Medical Library 37

Chapter 4 Medical Toys 41

Chapter 5 Medical Laboratory 49

Chpater 6 Diagnosis 67

Chapter 7 Healing Arts 81

Chapter 8 Pharmacy 113

Chapter 9 OB/GYN Homebirth 119

Chapter 10 *Materia Medica* 129

Chapter 11 Referrals to Specialists 321

Chapter 12 Insurance & Hospitals 327

Chapter 13 Public Health 333

References and Resources 337

Index............................. 347

About The Authors

Joel D. Wallach, BS, DVM, ND

Dr. Wallach has been involved in biomedical research and clinical medicine for 40 years. He received his B.S. Degree from the University of Missouri with a major in animal husbandry (nutrition) and field crops; a D.V.M. (veterinarian) from the University of Missouri; a three year post doctoral fellowship from the Center for the Biology of Natural Systems, Washington University; and an N.D. from the National College of Naturopathic Medicine, Portland, Oregon.

Dr. Wallach's research has resulted in the publication of more than 70 peer reviewed referred articles in the field of nutrition and pharmaceutical research; eight multi-author textbooks and authorship of a text/reference book on the subject of comparative medicine (W.B. Saunders Publishing Co., 1983).

Dr. Wallach's research in comparative medicine is based on more than 17,500 autopsy cases on 454 species of animals and 3,000 humans from the University of Missouri, Iowa State University, the Center for the Biology of Natural Systems, Washington University; the St. Louis Zoological Gardens; the Chicago Zoological Gardens; the Yerkes Regional Primate Research Center, Emory University, Atlanta, Georgia; the National College of Naturopathic Medicine, Portland, Oregon and Harbin Medical University, Harbin, Hei Long Jiang, People's Republic of China. He was a member of NIH site visit teams for four years and was a member of the 1968 NSF ad hoc committee that authored the 1968 Animal Welfare Act (humane housing and care of laboratory and captive exotic species); and Consulting Professor of Medicine, Harbin Medical University, Harbin, Hei Long Jiang,

People's Republic of China.

Dr. Wallach is an associate editor of *Quantum Medicine,* The Journal of the Association of Eclectic Physicians, and was the recipient of the 1988 Wooster Beach Gold Medal Award for a significant breakthrough in the basic understanding of the cause and pathophysiology of Cystic Fibrosis by the Association of Eclectic Physicians. He was nominated for a Nobel Prize in Medicine in 1991 for his work with the trace mineral selenium and its relationship to the congenital genesis of Cystic Fibrosis.

Dr. Wallach is the creator fo the 'Dead Doctors Don't Lie' tape, which sold more than 24 million copies and became the most listened to nutritional lecture in the history of the world!

Ma Lan, MD, MS

Dr. Ma Lan was educated in the People's Republic of China. Dr. Ma Lan received her M.D. from Beijing Medical University, took her residency in Peoples Hospital, Beijing and was a staff surgeon at the Canton Air Force Hospital. She received her M.S. (master of science) in transplant immunology from Zhong-Shan Medical University, Canton, People's Republic of China. As with all Chinese doctors, Dr. Ma Lan was educated in Traditional Chinese Medicine (i.e., acupuncture, herbs, manipulation, massage and hydrotherapy).

Dr. Ma Lan's research credits include being an exchange scholar at Harvard School of Medicine, Boston; a research fellow in laser microsurgery at St. Joseph's Hospital, Houston; the Department of Orthopaedic Microsurgery at the Medical College of Wisconsin, Milwaukee; and Department of Pharmacy, University of California, San Diego.

Dr. Ma Lan has eleven peer review publications to her credit in the fields of transplant immunology and microsurgery.

Lastly, Dr. Ma Lan was "sent to the countryside" for three years of hard labor during the "Cultural Revolution" of China, her crime "being an educated person and potentially dangerous to the revolution;" during these hard years, she was able to quietly be a doctor for a small farming village in the north of China using only Traditional Chinese Medicine.

Introduction

Drs. Wallach and Ma Lan are offering an educational as well as an entertaining manuscript in *Let's Play Doctor.*

Although alternative medicine holds quite a fascination for many of us, the subject when reviewed in its entirety, as this book does, can tend to become dreary reading. Not so here — with a wit deserving of wider recognition, the authors have succeeded in getting across information that allows the reader to grasp the importance of an idea without getting bored. Perhaps just as important, the reader is led into some serious discussions, without creating an impression that this is too deep or difficult for them to understand.

To bring the wealth of information from a veterinarian and naturopathic physician and a physician trained in Oriental medicine into a single volume has created a rare and fulfilling experience in the realm of wholism. Although the authors may give the impression of being slightly prejudiced as to their philosophy of healing, it is very obvious that these beliefs are based on facts and personal observations through many years of combined practice.

This is probably the first time a veterinarian turned physician has written about the similarities and discrepancies of treating animals as compared to humans. In some respects, it is frightening to know that the average animal that gets sick has a much better chance of getting well than humans do. That the food we humans eat is almost guaranteed to make animals sick, and that the minimum daily requirements for vitamins, minerals, proteins and fats are much more well researched in animals than man — and that the Recommended Daily Allowances are considerably lower than they should be.

When we consider that most animals live to approximately twenty times their age of maturity and man only five times his, we see the wisdom of a wellness lifestyle. *Let's Play Doctor* will guide you through the intricacies of basic health care, teach you how to supply your personal "health" cabinet and how to diagnose simple illnesses with ease. Enjoy reading the book!

— PETER HOLLIDAY &
JACKIE HOLLIDAY

Foreword

I have known Joel Wallach for many years and he never ceases to amaze me. He is busy, bright, and has his finger in more modalities of healing than I ever knew existed. I first met him about 23 years ago when I was getting started in the nutritional approach to the care and feeding of children. He was an inspiration as I was realizing how much the practice of veterinary medicine is like pediatrics: one really has to use one's diagnostic acumen to figure out the pathology.

I also became aware, with much help from Joel, that nutrition is the basis of health. He learned that through his veterinary training, and it was reinforced when he discovered that many of the diseases of animals have their counterparts in humans. He was able to show me that cystic fibrosis was related to the selenium deficiency of the mother during the pregnancy and that the full-blown disease in a child did not show up unless the deficiency was not corrected in the child early. Of course, the standard orthodox medical thought still believes that genetics and genetics alone determines who will get the disease and how seriously.

Joel has tried to get someone to believe his ideas are worth investigating, but once doctors make up their minds — well, you know how stubborn they can be. I was like that once, but people like Joel have helped me see the light. We (MD's) do not have all the answers. Knowing that he has been forced to deal with these negative attitudes despite his presentation of reproducible facts, you can understand his rather blatant doctor-bashing tirades scattered through the book. Some is fair, and some is overdone. Go for it, Joel, get it off your chest!

The nice thing about this book is that Joel assumes that the reader is reasonably intelligent. He assumes the reader knows what a rash is, and that if a person has a high fever and a convulsion, the reader would naturally dash off to the emergency room. Most everyone is aware that ice water is best for burns, not lard.

His background in Naturopathic Medicine makes his remedies credible. We need to become more familiar with the natural healing methods; we also need to know when to draw the line between home care and a real emergency. I can remember one of our children giving me a fright when she was but a baby. She had a high fever and a convulsion and I was trying to be calm. "Let me see, now, what do I tell people over the 'phone when they call about this problem — oh, yes, the comfortable hot bath to get the skin capillaries dilated, and then sponging off that red skin with a wash cloth so the water can evaporate." And it worked. We do need people around with some authority to tell us to do something when we become stoned, mute, and immobile when faced with the awesomeness of a medical, human condition that needs our ministrations.

Joel has put this book together so you can be a better and more efficient, caring, human being, mother, father, grandfather. You should be able to figure out what you can do at home and when you need some help from the doctor whose skills we recognize. We need books like Joel's to show us that alternative methods of health care are safe, cheap, and sometimes even more effective than drugs.

Thanks Joel, for bringing to our attention that we ourselves may be the best doctor for ourselves. After all, we live inside our own bodies; no-one else.

— **LENDON H. SMITH, MD**
5th September 1989

Preface

I am often accused of overzealous "ALLOPATH BASHING," but I prefer to call it justifiable homicide!!!

Will Rogers said, "If you need a good doctor get a veterinarian; animals can't tell him what's wrong, he's just got to know!" As a veterinarian involved in comparative medical research for 30 years, I have come to the conclusion that animals get a better deal when it comes to health care. The veterinary profession has raised the art and science of "preventive medicine" to its highest level by eliminating cancer, arthritis, liver disease, learning disabilities, birth defects, diabetes, muscular dystrophy, cystic fibrosis and dental diseases from laboratory, pet and farm animals. The "orthodox" medical profession's version of "preventive" medicine is vaccination!!! What is the "Magic Bullet" that the veterinarian has?

Preventive medicine is a matter of mind set. There are no third party carriers (insurance companies) for laboratory animals, pets and farm species. Why? Let's start with the farmer as that's where much of the basic research is done. Because of small profit margins, farmers and ranchers demand nutrition systems that prevent disease; they can't afford to have the vet come out twice each week for a calf that has a growth problem, birth defect or muscular dystrophy. Farmers and ranchers demand a hundred healthy calves for one hundred breeding cows that they are feeding and they expect the calves to reach market or reproductive age with little or no vet bills (this beats what we have come to expect as humans); just go to a zoo on a beautiful sunny Sunday and ask the first hundred women that go by if they have had any complicated pregnancies, children that were "delivered" by caesarean or children with birth defects and the results of your survey will blow your mind!

Farmers and ranchers are unwilling to pay for caesareans or pay for symptomatic therapies because they are working on a tight budget and the government does not have a Medicaid system for animals! "Preventive Medicine," veterinary style, is inexpensive and extremely effective in preventing the chronic diseases in animals that, if present, would make animal husbandry financially impossible. The American economic system of capitalism was allowed to take its course and the "money" was in finding a cheap and practical system of health care for animals — the result was preventive nutrition programs.

In contrast to the animal health systems, our human health systems are heavily supported by the government (clinical care as well as research) via legislation (i.e., Medicare, Medicaid, insurance, etc.). It is unfortunate that the mind set in human medicine is in treating the symptoms - this has produced a health care system that if union members learned that management and union stewards had reached such an agreement, they would wryly call it a "sweetheart deal" and call for a wildcat strike!!!

The United States government (FDA, NIH, legislation), the pharmaceutical industry (drug companies and the AMA have formed a "ménage á trois" or triangle that we choose to call the "Bermuda Triangle," "a black hole," a vortex out of control that sucks us all ever closer to destruction.

The "orthodox" medical system is an artificial system that depends on our government to survive. If it were left to the people, they will always choose a less formidable and less complex health care system. Under the protective and loving wing of the government, "orthodox" medicine has flourished as a house of cards.

Today the medical-pharmaceutical complex costs Americans more money each year than does all the military and Pentagon spending combined (i.e., $817 billion yet our health among the western industrialized nations is listed as 17th by the WHO). The extreme of this mentality is when "hungry orthodox" doctors get court orders to force you to take blood transfusions or take chemotherapy against your religious beliefs or charges you with child abuse and take your children away because your religion doesn't believe in vaccinations — is this not the same as forcing you to attend a state operated church???

It is of interest that the 10,000 year old system of Traditional Chinese Medicine only paid the doctor when you were well and stopped paying him when you became ill — this ancient system combined with the veterinary mind set would be an ideal medical system!!!

My personal experience with "orthodox" doctors both as my physicians and fellow researchers has been disastrous. The "orthodox" oncologist did not inform me of any alternatives when they "treated" my wife and killed her with chemotherapy in 1978; the "orthodox" doctors deemed my son to have "learning disabilities" when, in fact, he had severe and debilitating food allergies; pediatricians missed a diagnosis of folic acid deficiency anemia and a fractured arm in my children; and lastly, they killed my father with a nosocomial infection initiated during a very simple procedure. I am a faithful servant to anything I believe in so it took me until 1978 to realize that if I was to have a positive effect on human health I would have to go back to school and become a physician! I chose to become an N.D. (a naturopathic physician) because they believed philosophically in nutrition as a basic bulwark against disease. It is now time to share with you the accumulated knowledge of the veterinary profession and the naturopathic profession.

Lastly, the purpose of this book is to give you enough information so you can avoid unnecessary doctor or hospital visits. Most of us were normally curious about our bodies at an early age and we said to our friends, "Let's Play Doctor;" we "performed surgery," "delivered babies," gave "physicals" and wrote "prescriptions." As we grew older, we developed other interests (i.e., cars, math, dogs, etc.) and gleefully delegated our health care to the "orthodox" M.D. The government bureaucrats recognized a "good thing," ran to get in on the act and crowned the doctor "Bishops" of the "Bermuda Triangle" and themselves the first "Kings of the Realm."

Resist! Before you decide to follow your cardiologists advice, look in the obituaries for cardiologists who die under the age of fifty from a heart attack while jogging in the park! Let's Play Doctor together! Be like the proud little girl who said to her mother, "After we learned about the Boston Tea Party in school today, I threw all of the "orthodox" drugs from the medicine cabinet into the toilet."

"Praise the Lord and pass the herbs (ammunition)!"

—JOEL D. WALLACH, BS, DVM, ND

Chapter 1
Pre Med

"The medical profession is unconsciously irritated by lay knowledge."
— John Steinbeck

All "orthodox" doctors should be required to go to veterinary school as a pre-med course in the same way that Chinese doctors are required to complete training in Chinese Traditional Medicine before they enter into western type medical schools. The Chinese, who have a socialized medical system, realize that Chinese Traditional Medicine is a better buy for their money than western style "orthodox" medicine that is heavily tilted toward surgery, pharmaceuticals and hospitalization. In June 1989, I had the great honor to do a cystic fibrosis research project in China with several of the more famous Chinese physicians; while there I visited several CTM hospitals as well as their western style hospitals — it was wonderful. The CTM hospitals were teeming with patients, doctors and technicians performing acupuncture procedures, manipulation, hydrotherapy, physical therapy, etc. It looked like a railway station in a war zone full of evacuees of every description. Everyone was happy — even the patients who were packed as many as ten into a therapy room and hundreds waiting in the halls.

In contrast, the western type hospitals were politely filled with echoes of empty halls — the "orthodox" doctors get paid less than the CTM doctors and even less than cab drivers (I believe that's fair!).

The history of medicine reads like the history of nations in that there were, and still are, great battles going on, most of which are over "turf" (scope of practice) and raw materials (patients). At the time of Henry VIII (and for 10,000 years before), there was nothing uncommon in medical (herbal) expertise. Noblemen did in royal style what every household did out of necessity. In 1526, the first Herbal (medical self-help book) was translated from Greek and published for the common man. Those that followed were published by physicians and surgeons or chemists for consumption by their peers. Each author began to demand that everyone accept his collection of medications as the last word. The first government approved drug list was printed in Nuremberg between 1515 and 1544.

Paracelsus complained that physicians and apothecaries were pushing only exotic plants and forgetting those in the local "hedgerow" (they could get more for imported medicines than for the common backyard varieties even though in many cases the local herb was more effective) — the process had already begun!!! The full degree medical course at Cambridge in the 1500s took up to 14 years and was, therefore, the private domain of the wealthy (it was not uncommon for the medical students to take courses from schools in five to ten different countries in the process of getting their degree). During this time amateurs were the greatest competition to physicians and they complained loudly to the Parliament "for now every man without any study of necessary artes unto the knowledge of Physick will become a physician... every man, nay every wyfe will presume, not without mordre to many, to practyse Physick."

The early surgeons depended primarily on venereal

disease as their source of income (three out of four). Although the surgeons did not have a Guild or Charter, they fought bitterly with the Barber-Surgeons who had gotten a Royal Charter in 1462. The Barber-Surgeons were expected by charter to confine their efforts to cupping, bleeding, and tooth extraction. The apothecaries strongly believed they knew as much, or more, about medicine as did the physician. The chemist and apothecaries were expected by their charter to obtain medicines from the Royal Grocers' Company (food and drug company favored by the crown).

Now, in addition to all of these government approved practitioners, were the great masses of everyday people who dabbled in home self-help because the average man couldn't afford a Cambridge trained physician. The physicians complained "a great multitude of ignorant persons, of whom the greater part had no insight into physic, nor in any other kind of learning; some could not even read the letter on the book, so far forth, that common artificers, smiths, weavers and women, boldly and accustomedly took upon them great cures, to the high displeasure of God, great infamy of the faculty, and the grievous hurt, damage and destruction of many of the King's liege people."

In 1518, the College of Physicians was established and confirmed by Parliament to have medical control over the entire realm of England. In 1540, Parliament created several Acts which gave physicians control over Surgeons and Apothecaries. In a peacemaking offering to the unhappy Surgeons, Barbers were now forbidden to do surgery by the same Act. The Surgeons, in an all out effort to eliminate any competition in their now restricted scope of practice, set upon women herbalists and labeled them Witches. Because some of the Surgeons' victims of wrath had friends in Parliament, a new Act was passed that created a new type of recognized physician — the herbalist. The Act castigated the Surgeons for their greed and failure to treat the common man if they couldn't pay; "minding only their own lucre, and nothing the profit or ease of the diseased or patient, having sued, troubled and vexed divers honest persons, as well as men as women, whom God hath induced with the knowledge of nature, kind and operation of certain Herbs, Roots and Waters, and suing the ministering of them, to such as has been pained with customable diseases, as Women's Breasts being sore, a pin and the Web in the Eye, Uncomes of hands, scaldings, burnings, sore mouths, the stone, stagury, saucelim and morphew, and such other like diseases; and yet the said persons have not taken anything for their pains or cunnings, but have ministered the same to poor people only for neighbourhood and God's sake and pity and charity" (doesn't this sound somehow familiar — think of the fundraising efforts of a local village fire department to raise $500,000 for medical expenses to do a liver transplant on little Jimmy. The whole village gives of their charity but does the hospital or the "orthodox" doctor reduce the price? No! Little Jimmy must wait for his liver until the full "orthodox" medical fee is raised).

It is a sad fact that the "orthodox" medical profession worries more about competitors than they do about finding cures. Almost all "medical" discoveries were found by others than those "orthodox" doctors in universities and hospitals. For example, during the time when "orthodox" doctors believed that there was "spontaneous generation of life," Van Leeuwenhoek (a medical school janitor) discovered the microscope; Pasteur (a wine microbiologist) proved vaccines in animals, created rabies vaccine, determined that there were viral particles smaller than bacteria, and disproved the theory of spontaneous generation of life; Jenner (a country physician/veterinarian) noticed that milkmaids didn't get smallpox when they had cowpox sores on their hands so he protected his whole village by giving them cowpox! During this time, the physicians in the halls of the universities and hospitals fought against these new theories even to the point that Pasteur had to challenge them in the newspaper with a great sheep vaccination experiment in the outskirts of Paris (doesn't this sound like the media release of scientific "breakthroughs" of today?) — as we all know, Pasteur prevailed!

More recent was the discovery by veterinarians that ticks, flies and mosquitos transmitted tick fever to livestock and yellow fever to people; since Walter Reed was a physician and the head of the Panama Canal Health Committee, the hospital was named after him!

We know from military history and accelerated medical training programs that it doesn't take eight years to train a basic physician and another two to five years for residency and specialty training. Why then does the "orthodox" medical training take so long? It's elementary, Watson! It takes that long to totally enslave a young fertile mind to the "carrot" and "stick" system. Be good, write lots of prescriptions, refer lots of patients to the local hospital and you get the "carrot" (i.e., the Mercedes, big house, beach house, pool, investments, ski trips, golf every Wednesday, pretty wife, etc.). But woe unto you, Doctor; if you rebel in any way, you get the "stick" (i.e., you get your license jerked!).

The most blatant example of this "carrot" and "stick" system I know of is James Privitera, M.D. who was an early advocate of Laetrile (the alternative cancer medication). For his compassion to his terminal patients (you must know that Laetrile was legal in 23 states but not California because the "orthodox" oncologists had too strong of a lobby in the legislature), he was prosecuted by the State of California at the behest of the "orthodox" Medical Board, found guilty of using an "unauthorized" drug and thrown in jail. After great effort from the National Health Federation, Governor Jerry Brown pardoned Dr. Privitera. After his release, he returned to his practice, however, the events of his persecution had made him a west coast folk hero; the local doctors convinced the California authorities to continue their investigation of him to the point he wrote them a letter saying if they didn't cease and desist from harassment, he was going to hold a news conference and expose their tactics whereupon the good doctor was handcuffed, arrested and charged with extortion because he had "threatened" these United States! Something really stinks here! Fortunately, the local judge recognized that the "government had overreacted" and threw the case out of court! This judge should be a Supreme Court Justice!

"Orthodox"doctors are now advertising in the Yellow Pages and in newspapers, an act that would have brought down the "stick" upon them as recently as five years ago. What is happening? Well, it appears that despite the best efforts of physicians, the American people are beginning to shop around and look for a better way — forcing "orthodox" doctors to more openly fight for their share of the patient load! According to my good friend and colleague, William Moore, Esq. (who is a physician and attorney, a courtroom attorney in the classical Perry Mason terms), the fall of the "orthodox allopathic system" began in March of 1942 when the GI Bill of Rights was enacted at the same time that "orthodox" doctors were reaching their zenith in popularity, power and money.

The GI Bill created an education boom in the United States which is as much an antithesis to "orthodox" medicine as the Devil is to God!!! For the first time in the history of man, the patient had an equal or greater education than the doctor and/or a greater or equal financial portfolio than the doctor; patients ask questions today, want second opinions, shop around and refuse "elective procedures" (unnecessary operations). The "God-like" image of the "orthodox" doctor required total blind obedience and an educational stratification with himself at the top. This stratification doesn't exist anymore and we are no longer "hayseeds" to be dazzled into "buying the Brooklyn Bridge" (i.e., chemotherapy) or the "con man" (doctor) who charges you or your insurance $150 for a seven-minute visit or $2,000 for a physical.

Today, "orthodox" medicine is in its "agonal throes" (death struggle); all it needs for an appropriate euthanasia (mercy killing) or Coup de Grace is for the government to stop helping them — let the marketplace have its day; become your own "primary health care provider" (your grandmother did it!)

You need to make a conscious commitment and aggressively take over the responsibility for your own health for it is a great responsibility — yet, the rewards are great, too. You will not have to wait in a waiting room for hours while the doctor chats with a drug detail man or pinches his nurse. Use the time for aerobics or spend it with your family. The money you save in time, gas, parking fees (and parking tickets), unnecessary visits to your doctor and specialists, brand name drugs, extra clothes (nobody ever goes to the doctor in a raggedy housecoat), eating out, not to mention the doctor fees, will help you remodel your house, buy the Mercedes, buy the nice clothes, join a ritzy health club, and send the kids to college (your kids, not the "orthodox" doctors' kids!). You will know when you are committed because you will send back the visit reminder card with

People's Republic of China.

Dr. Wallach is an associate editor of *Quantum Medicine*, The Journal of the Association of Eclectic Physicians, and was the recipient of the 1988 Wooster Beach Gold Medal Award for a significant breakthrough in the basic understanding of the cause and pathophysiology of Cystic Fibrosis by the Association of Eclectic Physicians. He was nominated for a Nobel Prize in Medicine in 1991 for his work with the trace mineral selenium and its relationship to the congenital genesis of Cystic Fibrosis.

Dr. Wallach is the creator fo the 'Dead Doctors Don't Lie' tape, which sold more than 24 million copies and became the most listened to nutritional lecture in the history of the world!

keeps your clothes clean. "Scrub suits" (you know, the light green or blue cotton pajamas that doctors wear into surgery and the hospital lunch room — no wonder there are so many hospital infections — they get their spaghetti sauce into your surgical wound) and the lab coat can be worn to PTA meetings, grocery store and mechanic shop — see what additional respect and attention you get!!!

Chapter 2
Doctor Talk

> *"An unavoidable conclusion is that the way in which our medical care system has evolved has created conditions that increase the likelihood of damage to the patient."*
>
> — Rick Carlson
> *The End of Medicine*

The language of medicine is a jealously guarded secret of the Guild of "orthodox" doctors. It is a way that they can communicate with each other in our presence and only they know what is being said. It's kind of a medical "pig-Latin" to be used by the "in group," sort of a carry-over from their campus fraternity days. This medical "pig-Latin" is used on hospital records, medical records, insurance forms, laboratory reports, letters of referral and in prescription writing. It is our intention to give you a crash course in the basic fundamentals of "doctor talk" so that you can translate your own medical records and prescriptions.

Most medical language is derived from Latin or Greek and has been rendered down to abbreviations (Table 2-1), prefixes (Table 2-2), and suffixes (Table 2-3). The original words have been abbreviated to save space on records; it also makes it impossible for you to get the original meaning of the word. In fact, the hardest "hurdle" to jump or "hoop" to jump through in any healing art pre-med program is the learning of the "doctor talk."

Prefixes are simply modifiers of words; for example, the word "tension" infers pressure but without a medical prefix it is of little value. The prefix "hyper-" placed before the word tension gives "hypertension" which is equated to high blood pressure. The same word "tension" can be modified by the prefix "hypo" which translates to low blood pressure. All medical prefixes are used in the same manner. Table 2-2 is a basic guide to the more commonly used prefixes. If you have an unusual medical condition with unique language you will need to use the medical dictionary (don't be bashful — your specialist does, too!).

Medical suffixes work in much the same manner as prefixes in that they modify the word to which they are applied. A good example is the suffix "-emia" meaning blood. The prefix "a" or "an" by itself means "without;" add the suffix "-emia" and you have "anemia" or "without blood." Another example would be the word parasite. Add the suffix "-emia" and you have "parasitemia" or parasite infestation in the blood (i.e., malaria, filariasis, etc.).

Medical records normally contain several sections including : MEDICAL HISTORY back to great grandma's diabetes, your childhood diseases and your past prescriptions, etc. REVIEW OF ORGAN SYSTEMS deals in more detail with chronic problems with your liver, heart, lungs, etc. HISTORY OF CURRENT ILLNESS covers in detail why you are in the doctor's office for the current visit. PHYSICAL is the "orthodox" doctor's way of laying on hands and directly, or indirectly, examining many organ systems.

The physical exam should include the blood pressure, pulse, temperature, weight as well as a detailed inspection of all external and all reachable internal organ systems. Very frequently a doctor will want to have his nurse collect blood, urine and fecal samples to send to the laboratory for additional indirect evaluation of an organ or organ system. The physical and lab can be very expensive, costing from $350 to $500. In addition, the time expenditure of taking your detailed history, waiting at all the stations for the doctor or nurse can cost you in time from four hours to a full eight hour day.

It should be obvious to you by now that (except for extraordinary cases) most of the information accumulated by the doctor comes from you and that you can keep your own organized records in a loose-leaf notebook or in a 5x8 card file. An example of simple home use history record is given in Figure 2-1.

Prescriptions are another area of great interest to us (if they are incorrect they can kill you!!!) yet, they are virtually impossible to translate without knowledge of the basic language or format. The typical prescription (Table 2-4) is a coded message from the "orthodox" doctor to the pharmacist (apothecary) giving instructions as to which medicine should be dispensed to you including brand, doses, number of doses, etc. A typical prescription contains four basic parts:

1) Superscription — the patient's name, address, age, date.

2) Inscription — the name of the prescribed drug, dose form (i.e., capsule, tablets, liquid, etc.) and the amount of drug per dose.

3) Subscription — mixing instructions and/or the number of doses to be dispensed.

4) Signature — which are the instructions to the

patient that the doctor wants placed on the bottle or box. The doctor's name, address, and telephone number are placed in this section and may include the DEA number if the prescription is a narcotic. An example of a typical prescription is found in Figure 2-2.

Medical measurements are often unique and not used anywhere else or may be of metric values infrequently used in the average American life. These measurements are given to you in easy conversion tables (Table 2-5). Medical measurements are used by the doctor, pharmacist, hospital, laboratories and drug companies. A serious knowledge of these measurements are absolutely essential if you are going to be responsible for your own health care as the "primary health care provider" (the insurance term given to your family doctor or internist).

Terms for herbal function (Table 2-6) and herbal preparations (Table 2-7) have carried over into drug terminology; knowledge of these terms is essential as they are required tools for use of the PDR (Physicians Desk Reference). Isn't it interesting that drug dealers in "illicit drugs" use "beepers" and the same terminology and metric system (i.e., "Kilos") as the "dealers" of "legal drugs?"

Lastly, if you are going to be up on "doctor talk" you need to learn the rules and terms for golf, boating, skiing and investments. Doctors don't carry their "beepers" to their Wednesday jaunt to the golf course anymore (it isn't good form!). An "orthodox" doctor without a broker is like "a day without sunshine!"

Figure 2-1. "Playing Board" for "Family Practice"

Name ____________________ Wt. ________ Height ________ DOB ________

Medical History ____

Medications ____

BP ____________ Pulse ____________ Temp ____________ Hair ______ Eyes ________

Skin & Nails ____________ Ears ____________ Reflexes ____________

Mouth ____________ Tongue ____________ Lymph Nodes ____________

Genitals ____________ Breast ____________ Chest ____________

Lungs ____________ Heart ____________ Abdomen ____________

Bones ____________ Anus/Rectum ____________ Prostate ____________

Vagina/Cervix ____________

Lab:

Blood ____________ Urine ____________ Stool ____________ Hair ____________

Special Notes

Figure 2-2. Prescription Format

Jane A. Doe 32 y o a May 25, 1989
1234 Homestead
Independence , Missouri
63114

VALIUM, Tab., 5 mg ad lib
30 tabs

Sig. 5 mg Valium ad lib for nerves

I. Atro Genic, M. D.
ORTHODOX CLINIC
Gotcha, USA

Table 2-1: Medical Abbreviations and Symbols

AAA	abdominal aortic aneurysm
A.A.	Associate of Arts degree
ABG	arterial blood gasses
ACE	adrenal cortical extract
ACTH	adrenocorticotropic hormone
ADH	antidiuretic hormone
ADL	activities of daily living
ADP	adenosine diphosphate
ALL	acute lymphoblastic leukemia
AMA	American Medical Association
AML	acute myelocytic leukemia
AODM	adult-onset diabetes mellitus
AP	angina pectoris
ARF	acute renal failure
As	arsenic
ASA	aspirin (acetylsalicylic acid)
ASHD	arteriosclerotic heart disease
ASO	arteriosclerosis obliterans
ASO	antistreptolysin O (titer)
ATP	adenosine triphosphate
AVM	arteriovenous malformation
B.A.	Bachelor of Arts degree
BAL	British anti-lewisite
BCG	Bacillus Calmette — Guerin (vaccine)
b.i.d	two times a day
BMR	basal metabolic rate
BP	blood pressure
BPH	benign prostatic hypertrophy
B.S.	Bachelor of Science degree
BSA	body surface area
BSP	sulfobromophthalein
BUN	blood urea nitrogen

Table 2-1: Medical Abbreviations and Symbols (Continued)

BX	biopsy
C	carbon; Celsius; centigrade; complement
CA	cancer
Ca	calcium
CAD	coronary artery disease
CAH	chronic active hepatitis
CALD	chronic active liver disease
CBC	complete blood count
CBD	common bile duct
CC	chief complaint
c.c.	cubic centimeter
CCK	cholecystokinin
CCU	coronary care unit
Cd	cadmium
CDE	common duct exploration
CF	cystic fibrosis
CF	compliment fixation
Ch.	chapter
CHD	coronary heart disease
CHF	congestive heart failure
Ci	curie
Cl	chloride
cm	centimeter
Cn	cyanide
CNS	central nervous system
Co	cobalt
CO	carbon monoxide
CO	cardiac output
C/O	complaints of
CO_2	carbon dioxide
COPD	chronic obstructive pulmonary disease

Table 2-1: Medical Abbreviations and Symbols (Continued)

CP	cerebral palsy
CPK	creatine phosphokinase
CPR	cardiopulmonary resuscitation
Cr	chromium
CRF	chronic renal failure
CSF	cerebrospinal fluid
CT	computed tomography
Cu	copper
cu mm	cubic millimeter
CVA	cerebrovascular accident
CVP	central venous pressure
D.C.	chiropractic physician
D & C	dilation & curettage
D/C	discontinue
D.D.S.	dentist
DIC	disseminated intravascular coagulation
DIP	distal interphalangeal joint
DJD	degenerative joint disease
DKA	diabetic ketoacidosis
dl	deciliter
DM	diabetes melitis
DMSO	dimethyl sulfoxide
DNA	deoxyribonucleic acid
D.O.	osteopathic physician
DOA	dead on arrival
DOE	dyspnea on exertion
D.Sc.	Doctor of Science
DPT	diphtheria/pertussis/tetanus
DU	duodenal ulcer
D.V.M.	veterinarian
D/W	dextrose in water
D5W	dextrose 5% in water

Table 2-1: Medical Abbreviations and Symbols (Continued)

DX	diagnosis
E	Earth
ECF	extracellular fluid
ECG	electrocardiogram (EKG)
ECT	electric convulsive therapy
EDTA	ethylene diamine tetraacetic acid
EEG	electroencephalogram
EFA	essential fatty acids
ENT	ear, nose and throat
EENT	eye, ear, nose and throat
EPA	eicosapentanoic acid
ESR	erythrocyte sedimentation rate
F	Fahrenheit
FBS	fasting blood sugar
FDA	Food & Drug Administration
FFA	free fatty acids
ft	feet (or foot measurement)
FFT	failure to thrive
FUO	fever of unknown origin
Fx	fracture
GB	gall bladder
GE	gastroenteritis
GI	gastrointestinal
gm	gram
G-6-PD	glucose-6-phosphate dehydro.
GTF	glucose tolerance factor
GTT	glucose tolerance test
GU	genitourinary
GYN	gynecology
h	hour
HA	headache
Hb	hemoglobin (or Hgb)
HBP	high blood pressure

Table 2-1: Medical Abbreviations and Symbols (Continued)

HCI	hydrochloric acid
HCO_3	bicarbonate
Hct	hematocrit
Hg	mercury
HI	hemagglutination inhibition
HLA	human leukocyte group A
H_2O	water
H_2O_2	hydrogen peroxide
HPI	history of present illness
HPT	hyperparathyroidism
HTN	hypertension
Hx	history
Hz	hertz (cyles per second)
I	iodine
ICF	intracellular fluid
ICU	intensive care unit
ID	intradermal
IDA	iron deficiency anemia
IHD	ischemic heart disease
IHSS	idiopathic hypertrophic subaortic stenosis
IgA	immunoglobulin A (IgG; IgM)
IM	intramuscular
IMP	impression
IP	intraperitoneal
IPPB	inspiratory positive pressure breathing
IU	international unit
IV	intravenous
IVP	intravenous pyelogram
IVC	inferior vena cava
J	joule
K	potassium

Table 2-1: Medical Abbreviations and Symbols (Continued)

Kcal	kilocalorie (food calories)
KD	kidney disease
Kg	kilogram
17-KGS	17-ketogenic steroids
17-KS	17-ketosteriods
KUB	kidney, ureter and bladder
L	liter
l	left
lb	pound
LBP	low back pain
LDH	lactic dehydrogenase
LD50	lethal dose 50 (50% fatal dose)
LE	lupus erythematosus
LFT	liver function test
LLQ	lower left quadrant
LMD	local medical doctor
LPN	licensed practical nurse
LUQ	left upper quadrant
M	molar
m	meter
mCi	millicurie
MCH	mean corpuscular hemoglobin
MCHC	mean corpuscular hemoglobin conc.
MCT	medium chain triglycerides
MCV	mean corpuscular volume
MD	muscular dystrophy
M.D.	physician
MDR	minimum daily requirement
MEq	milliequivalent
Mg	magnesium
mg	milligram
MI	mitral insufficiency; myocardial infarction

Table 2-1: Medical Abbreviations and Symbols (Continued)

MIC	minimum inhibitory concentration
min	minute
mIU	milli-international unit
ml	milliliter
MLD	minimum lethal dose
mM	millimole
mm	millimeter
Mn	manganese
mo	month
MOM	milk of magnesia
mol wt	molecular weight
mOsm	milliosmol
MRC	Medical Research Council
MS	multiple sclerosis; mitral stenosis
M.S.	Master of Science degree
N	nitrogen
Na	sodium
NAD	no apparent distress
NCI	National Cancer Institute
N.D.	naturopathic physician
NG	nasogastric
ng	nanogram
NIH	National Institutes of Health
nm	nanometer
NPO	nothing by mouth
NRC	National Research Council
NSF	National Science Foundation
NTS	nontropical sprue
N & V	nausea and vomiting
O	oxygen
O_2	oxygen gas

Table 2-1: Medical Abbreviations and Symbols (Continued)

OB	obstetrics
OB/GYN	obstetrics & gynecology
OBS	organic brain syndrome
OD	overdose
17-OHCS	17-hydroxycorticosteroids
OHD	organic heart disease
OR	operating room
OT	occupational therapy
OTC	over-the-counter (drugs)
oz	ounce
P	phosphorus; pressure
PA	pernicious anemia
PAME	preanasthesia medical exam
PAN	periarteritis nodosa
PAO_2	alveolar oxygen pressure
PAT	paroxysmal artrial tachycardia
Pb	lead
PBI	protein bound iodine
PCM	protein calorie malnutrition
PCO_2	carbon dioxide pressure
pH	acidity scale
Ph.d.	doctor of philosophy
PID	pelvic inflammatory disease
PND	paroxysmal nocturnal dyspnea
PO2	venous oxygen pressure
ppd	purified protein derivative (tuberculin)
ppm	parts per million
p.r.n.	as needed
PS	pulmonary stenosis
psi	pounds per square inch
PSP	phenolsulfonphthalein
pt	patient

Table 2-1: Medical Abbreviations and Symbols (Continued)

PT	physical therapy
PTA	prior to admission
PU	peptic ulcer
PVC	premature ventricular contraction
PVD	peripheral vascular disease
qd	every day
qh	every hour
q.i.d.	4 times daily
q2h	every 2 hours
q.s.	quantity sufficient
R/r	roentgen (measure of radiation)
RA	rheumatoid arthritis
rbc	red blood cell
RDA	recommended daily allowance
RES	reticuloendothelial system
RF	rheumatic fever
RHD	rheumatic heart disease
RLQ	right lower quadrant
R.N.	registered nurse
RNA	ribonucleic acid
R/O	rule out
RoRx	radiation therapy
ROS	review of symptoms
RUQ	right upper quadrant
Rx	take thee of (prescription)
S	sulfur
SAH	subarachnoid hemorrhage
SaO_2	arterial oxygen saturation
SBE	subacute bacterial endocarditis
SBO	small bowel obstruction
sc	subcutaneous
Se	selenium

Table 2-1: Medical Abbreviations and Symbols (Continued)

SGOT	serum glutamic oxaloacetic transaminase
SGPT	serum glutamic pyruvic transaminase
SIDS	sudden infant death syndrome
SLE	systemic lupus erythematosus
SOB	shortness of breath
S/P	status postoperative
sp gr	specific gravity
sq	square
sq m	square meter
STS	serologic test for syphilis
STSG	split thickness skin graft
SVCO	superior vena cava obstruction
Sx	symptoms
T & A	tonsillectomy & adenoidectomy
TB	tuberculosis
tbsp	tablespoon
TCE	transitional cell epithelioma
TEF	tracheoesophageal fistula
TG	triglycerides
THA	total hip arthroplasty
THC	transhepatic cholangiogram
TI	tricuspid insufficiency
TIA	transient ischemic attacks
t.i.d.	3 times per day
TKA	total knee arthroplasty
TLA	translumbar aortogram
TMJ	temporomandibular joint
TPN	total parenteral nutrition
tsp	teaspoon
TUR	transurethral resection
U/u	unit

Table 2-1: Medical Abbreviations and Symbols (Continued)

U/A	urine analysis
UGI	upper gastrointestinal
URI	upper respiratory infection
USDA	U.S. Department of Agriculture
USPHS	U.S. Public Health Service
UTI	urinary tract infection
V & P	vagotomy & pyloroplasty
VH	vaginal hysterectomy
VS	vital signs
wbc	white blood cells
WDHA	watery diarrhea, hypokalemia achlorhydria
WHO	World Health Organization
wk	week
WNL	within normal limits
wt	weight
yr	year
ZE	Zollinger-Ellison (syndrome)

TABLE 2-2. Common Medical Prefixes

Prefix	Meaning	Prefix	Meaning
a- or an-	without	hypo-	too little
cardi-	heart	myel-	marrow
chol-	bile	nephr-	kidney
col-	colon	neur-	nerve
cyst-	bladder	oste-	bone
enter-	intestine	poly-	many
gastr-	stomach	proct-	anus, rectum
hepat-	liver	pseudo-	false
hydr-	water	pulm-	lung
hyper-	too much		

TABLE 2-3. Common Medical Suffixes

Suffix	Meaning
-algia	pain
-clysis	drenching
-cyte	cell
-ectomy	excision
-emia	in the blood
-genic or -genesis	formation
-gnosis	knowledge
-itis	inflammation
-lytic or -lysis	destruction
-malacia	softening
-opia	vision
-pathy	disease of
-phagia	eating
-phobia	fear of
-pnea	breath
-privia or -penia	poverty of; without
-ptosis	dropped; fallen
-sclerosis	hardening
-scopy	inspection
-stenosis	narrowing
-stomy	mouth; new opening
-trophy	nutrition; growth
-uria	urine

Table 2-4. Terminology for Prescription Reading

Abbreviation	Latin	Meaning
aa	ana	of each
ac	ante cibum	before meals
ad lib	ad libitum	as needed
alt dieb	alternis diebus	every other day
alt hor	alternis horis	every other hour
alt noc	alternis noctibus	every other night
b.i.d.	bis in die	twice each day
c	cum	with
contin	continuetur	let it be continued
dil	dilutus	dilute
div	divide	divide
fl	fluidus	fluid
h	hora	hour
hd	hor decubitus	at bedtime
hs	hor somni	at sleeping time
m et n	mane et nocte	morning and night
nb	nota bene	note well
od	omni die	daily
om	omni mane	every morning
on	omni nocte	every night
part vic	partibus vicibus	in divided doses

Table 2-4. Terminology for Prescription Reading (Continued)

pc .... post cibum .... after food

prn .... pro re nata .... as required

pulv .... pulvis .... powder

qd .... quaque die .... every day

qh .... quaque hora .... every hour

q 2 h .... quaque sec hora ...... every 2 hours

q 3 h .... quaque ter hora ...... every 3 hours

q.i.d. .... quater in die .... four times each day

qs .... quantum sufficit ..... as much as is sufficient

Rx .... recipe .... take

S or sig .... signa .... give following directions

s .... sign .... without

sos .... si opus sit .... if necessary

ss .... semis .... one half

stat .... statim .... at once

t.i.d. .... ter in die .... three times each day

TABLE 2-5. Medical Weights & Volumes

60 drops (gtt)	= 1 teaspoon (tsp)
3 teaspoonfuls	= 1 tablespoon (tbsp)
2 tablespoonfuls	= 1 fluid ounce
6 fluid ounces	= 1 teacupful
8 fluid ounces	= 1 cupful/1 glassful

1 drop	= 1 minim	= 0.06 ml
1 tsp	= 1 fluid dram	= 5.0 ml
1 tbsp	= 4 fluid drams	= 15.0 ml
2 tbsp	= 1 fluid ounce	= 30.0 ml
1 teacupful	= 6 fluid ounces	=180.0 ml
1 glassful	= 8 fluid ounces	=240.0 ml

1000 ml (1 liter)	= 1 quart (1.10119 liters)
500 ml	= 1 pint (550.599 ml)
240 ml	= 8 fluid ounces
30 ml	= 1 fluid ounce (28.412 ml)
15 ml	= 4 fluid drams
4 ml	= 1 fluid dram
1 ml	= 15 minims
0.06 ml	= 1 minim (1 drop)

1000 gm (kilogram)	= 2.2 pounds
454 gm	= 1 pound
30 gm	= 1 ounce (31.1 gm)
15 gm	= 4 drams
6 gm	= 90 grains
1 gm	= 15 grains
1000 mg	= 1 gm
60 mg	= 1 grain
1 mg	= 1000 mcg

TABLE 2-6. Terms of Herbal Function

TERM	FUNCTION
Alternative	produce healthful change
Anodyne	pain relief
Anthelmintic	expel worms or parasites
Antiemetic	stops vomiting
Antiphlogistic	reduces inflammation
Antiseptic	stop or prevent sepsis (infection)
Antispasmodic	reduces spasms
Aperient	mild laxative
Aphrodisiac	sexual stimulant
Aromatic	arrests discharges
Astringent	constricting or binding
Cardiac	heart tonic
Carminative	relieves gas in GI tract
Cathartic	purgative
Cephalic	used for head ailments
Cholagogue	increases bile flow
Demulcent	soothes mucus membranes
Depurative	cleansing
Dermatic	agent for dermatitis
Diaphoretic	increases perspiration
Digestive	aids digestion
Diuretic	increase urination
Emetic	induces vomiting
Emmenagogue	induces menstruation
Emollient	agent that softens
Expectorant	induces productive coughing
Febrifuge	abates fevers
Hemostatic	stops bleeding
Hepatic	remedy for liver diseases
Herpetic	remedy for skin eruptions
Hydragogue	remedy for moving water

TABLE 2-6. Terms of Herbal Function (Continued)

Term	Function
Hypnotic	induces sleep or relaxation
Irritant	induces a local inflammation
Laxative	induces bowel function
Lithontriptic	dissolves urinary calculi
Mucilaginous	soothing to inflamed parts
Mydriatic	dilates pupil
Myotic (miotic)	contracts pupil
Narcotic	induces stupor or sleep
Nauseant	induces vomiting
Nervine	sedative for the nerves
Nutritive	nourishing properties
Ophthalmicum	remedy for eye diseases
Oxytocic	induces uterine contractions
Parturient	promotes labor
Purgative	induces evacuation of bowels
Refrigerant	agent that cools
Resolvent	dissolves tumors
Rubefacient	increases circulation
Sedative	quiets nerves
Sialagogue	induces increased salivation
Sternutatory	induces sneezing
Stimulant	induces increased function
Stomachic	increases stomach digestion
Styptic	topical agent to stop bleeding
Sudorific	induces perspiration
Taeniafuge	agent that expels tapeworms
Tonic	increases strength or tones
Vermifuge	agent that expels parasites (roundworms)
Vulnerary	agent that induces wound healing

TABLE 2-7. Terms of Herbal Preparation Technique

INFUSION:	Pour one pint of boiling water over one ounce of dried herb and let it stand for 1/2 hour. Strain off clear supernate. Dose is normally one tablespoon to a teacupful t.i.d.
DECOCTION:	Place one ounce of dried herb in 1 1/2 pints of cold water and boil for 20-30 minutes. Strain off clear supernate. Dose is one tablespoon to one ounce of water t.i.d.
TINCTURE:	One to two ounces of dried herbs are steeped in one pint of grain alcohol (brandy or vodka) for two days with vigorous shaking t.i.d. The decoction is strained and one tablespoon of the clear liquid is used t.i.d.
CAPSULE:	The herb is powdered and then placed in a two-piece gelatin capsule. The capsule may be added to hot water for tea, opened and made into paste for poultices, tinctures, decoctions, infusions or swallowed.
TABLET:	The dried herb is pressed into a tablet shape with an excipient (binder or carrier). The tablet can be used in all the same ways that a capsule can.

Chapter 3
Medical Library

"The Chinese character for "crisis" is made up of two different characters, one signifying "danger" and the other "opportunity."

— Jacob Needleman

No medical practice including your home "doctor's office" would be complete without a basic medical library. This book is kept at a reasonable cost by not repeating information better gotten from other sources. A basic home medical library should include a medical dictionary — our personal choice being the Dorlands Medical Dictionary published by W.B. Saunders Publishing Company (the largest medical publishing company in the world). This book is an excellent source of complete definitions and for details of anatomy (i.e., skeleton, muscles, viscera, nerves, cardiovascular system, endocrine system and lymphatic system).

A second must for the home medical library is the classic Merck Manual which lists all currently important human diseases in the United States and Europe. This book gives a complete picture of the disease from cause, incubation, symptoms, projected outcome, "orthodox" treatment and common complications. The value of this book is multiple, including helping list diseases that cause certain symptoms and "rule-in" or "rule-out" diseases that you think you might have. Another value of the Merck Manual is that it is the epitome of "orthodox" medicine in approach to diagnosis and treatment. When your doctor used to excuse himself during a physical or consultation, he was probably going to his office library to "consult" the Merck Manual to feverishly search for a diagnosis or to find out which diagnostic test to run on you!!!

The PDR (Physicians Desk Reference) is an excellent resource book. It lists all drugs approved by the FDA including chemical composition, mode of action, indications, contraindications and manufacturer. The PDR is printed yearly as a new editions so the previous years edition can be purchased from any used bookstore. If you are "hooked" to an "orthodox" MD, this book is a must — it will save your life! Most MDs do not refer to this book as often as they should and as a result nearly 40% of all hospitalizations are the result of iatrogenic disease (doctor caused). I have seen in my practice literally hundreds of patients that came to me with shopping bags full of medication — most of the medications were to counter the side effects of the original medications!!!

I (Wallach) was once an expert witness in a case where an ND was being tried for wrongful death and injury to a patient in Fayetteville, NC. The state contended that the ND killed the patient with her therapies (although the patient died in a VA hospital some six months after his last visit to the ND). A review of the terminal records showed that the VA hospital had used no less then eleven pain killers and sedatives without reducing the dosage of any of them!!! No one on the VA hospital staff had taken the time to read the PDR — they killed this man with an overdose of medications and were trying to slip the blame on the ND. The jury found the ND not guilty to the charges!!!

Specialty books on therapies and diseases that you

might have are useful. These books are what separates a "specialist" from a "general practitioner." Some of the most useful references are "booklets" that have already condensed a lot of the information for you from ten thick texts into 25 pages of concentrated and useful information. If you are going to use particular "modalities" (treatment methods) such as herbology, homeopathy, acupuncture, reflexology or kinesiology, you will want one or more of the complete "pharmacopeias" or "how to" books for more detail — again, this book would become a 1000-page "tome" that would have an exorbitant cost (i.e., $120 like most medical text books) which would keep Let's Play Doctor out of the hands of the masses.

Lastly, every "medical library" should have one or more periodicals (i.e., monthly or quarterly). The periodicals should take the form of one or more health-oriented magazines or journals. Specialty periodicals of every disease, exercise and therapy are available if you are interested in expanding your library's value. We also suggest a subscription of *USA TODAY* as they review the orthodox medical literature for interesting health breakthroughs which will keep you up to date.

Videos and audio cassettes are available on just about every medical subject from disease to therapy. These are available commercially and may be listened to or viewed at your closest medical school library — they are all state and U.S. government supported and are, therefore, required to give you free access. Also use your audio tapes in your car tape deck — just like the "orthodox" doctors do on their way to the golf course!!!

Chapter 4
Medical Toys

"An American Medical Association publication for doctors relates a tale of an engineer who was called in by a doctor whose electrocardiograph was not recording the heart action of a patient. The technician came promptly. He started to check at the electrical outlet and worked back slowly to the connection to the patient in the next room and found the patient dead. No one had even noticed that the patient's heart itself had stopped."

— Arthur S. Freese

Instruments and equipment used by doctors are referred to as "toys" because "orthodox" doctors have a lot of fun with these instruments and after awhile tire of them and look for newer and better equipment to "play" with. The old saying that "the only difference between men and boys is the price of their toys" holds true for "orthodox" doctors — "the only difference between a general practitioner and a specialist is the price of their toys!!!"

One of the "privileges" of a hospital association for the "orthodox" doctor is a lower overhead. In other words, he can use the hospital surgery room, x-ray equipment and nursing staff support without having to pay for it himself (it would be like a mechanic using all the diagnostic equipment and tools in a Sears Automotive Shop and keeping all of his fees; Sears would bill the customer separately for use of the shop space, tools and consumable materials). Compare this with a veterinarian who must have the x-ray equipment, surgery room, orthopedic equipment, obstetrical equipment, dental equipment, pharmacy, etc.!!! Why are "orthodox" doctors so much more expensive than veterinarians — it must be the pressure to make their Mercedes payment and their greens fees!!!

In keeping with the concept of Let's Play Doctor, there are some basic "toys" (instruments) that are required to "play the game." It is of great benefit to all of us that many of the basic "toys" used by "orthodox" doctors in the "practice" of medicine are sold at pharmacies and variety stores at very reasonable prices. Slightly more sophisticated equipment may be purchased at college bookstores and medical and laboratory supply houses.

The thermometer is as basic a medical "toy" as you can get. There are two basic types. The oral thermometer is used to measure the core body temperature — an elevated temperature or "fever" is usually indicative of an infection (bacterial, viral or fungus) or active invasive or degenerative disease process (i.e., rheumatoid arthritis, cancer, liver cirrhosis, etc.).

Marked variations in basal body temperature can be associated with normal body function (i.e., ovulation). Subnormal basal body temperature can be a useful sign to determine the status of your thyroid gland (i.e., too low means a "hypo" thyroid condition — you see it doesn't take too long to learn "doctor" talk). Normal temperature reading for the oral thermometer are 98.6°F or 37°C.

The rectal thermometer is especially useful for infants and patients with oro-facial disease that makes the use of the oral thermometer impossible. Normal temperature readings for the rectal thermometer are 101.2°F or 38.5°C.

A good light source such as a penlight, flashlight or illuminated head loop is useful for looking at the throat, nose, eyes (i.e., pupil reaction to light) and for lighting a "surgical field" (i.e., removal of splinters, debris from abrasions, etc).

The reflex hammer is used to check the knee and elbow reflexes. This test gives you an impression of the status of the spinal cord and nerves. Back injuries or any pressure on the spinal cord will affect the reflexes. Right and left side reflexes should be equal in intensity. Absence of the reflex on either side is a signal to seek professional help (i.e., chiropractor, naturopathic physician, etc.).

A watch with a second hand or a good digital watch with running seconds is useful for monitoring the pulse, respiratory rate and test times for a variety of home "lab" tests. There are watches with a sensor that count your pulse for you if you find it difficult to locate your pulse. Athletes will have a pulse rate in the 50+ range while the average pulse ranges from 65 to 80. Elevated pulses occur with fever, cardiovascular disease, pulmonary disease, anemia, pain and food allergies.

The respiratory rate averages ten to twelve per minute. Elevated rates indicate cardiovascular disease, lung disease, anemia, fever or pain.

The sphygmomanometer or "blood pressure cuff" is a very useful "toy" and can be mastered by a child very quickly. To make this "toy" work, you will need a stethoscope. Blood pressure readings consist of two parts. A typical BP reading is 125/80 mm Hg. The first number (125) is the pressure in the arteries during the contraction of the heart (systolic pressure) and the second number (80) is the pressure in the arteries during the relaxation of the heart (diastolic pressure). Elevations in the BP above 140 on the systolic phase and/or 90 on the diastolic phase indicate "hyper"tension (you see — there goes "doctor" talk again) or high BP.

An ophthalmoscope/otoscope combination is in order for those with serious interests in "playing doctor." This instrument can be used as a light source and will allow direct views of the inner ear, eardrum, ear canal (i.e., arteriosclerosis, diabetes, copper deficiencies, hemorrhage from injury, cataracts, etc.).

"Surgical" instruments or "toys" such as thumb forceps (tweezers), scissors, hemostats, needle holders, suture needles and even fingernail clippers and tape are invaluable. The removal of splinters, sutures (stitches), debris from abrasions, removal of "hangnails" and flaps of dead and torn skin can be done at home by the most inexperienced of "surgeons." Closure of lacerations (cuts) can be done with butterfly bandages or wound strips.

The more aggressive "surgeon" can procure and use silk suture with "swagged-on" needles (needles that are precrimpted onto suture material — this configuration reduces the size of the hole in the skin created by pulling the needle and thread through the skin). You will need topical local anesthetic (i.e., acupuncture or xylocaine) and needle holders (a special surgical clamp used to grip the small suture needle while making "stitches").

The sterilization of all "surgical" instruments or "toys" is paramount. Boiling in distilled water for 30 minutes is a very economical and acceptable technique. The sterilized "toys" can be placed in zip lock "boiling" baggies for sterilization and storage to prevent contamination.

Sterile rubber gloves are multi-useful and disposable

supplies that can be purchased at your local pharmacy. They can be worn while examining the prostate or rectum for hemorrhoids, while examining the vagina and cervix or can be used by the "surgeon" while placing "stitches," performing "surgery" or protect the "doctor" while treating infectious skin diseases (i.e., boils, impetigo and abscesses).

Syringes are useful for B-12 and other vitamin shots as well as for autoimmune urine therapy, irrigating abscesses and contaminated wounds.

A balance-type scale to monitor weight is useful for growth rates in children, self-control weight loss programs, sudden weight gain (i.e., dropsy, diabetes, toxemia of pregnancy, etc.).

Those individuals who are involved in a lot of rigorous athletic activities will want a tuning fork to test for fractures. A "C" tuning fork is recommended. If an injury to a limb or digit occurs and is suspected to be a fracture, get the tuning fork vibrating by rapping it against the palm of your hand and place the stem over the sensitive area. If a fracture is present (even a hairline fracture), the tuning fork will create a burning pain. If there is no fracture, no difference will be noted.

Larger "toys" may be purchased new from college bookstores and used from college bulletin boards or garage sales. Microscopes are useful for doing your own CBC and "differential," examining "stool" samples (bowel movement) for parasite eggs, determining types of bacteria or fungus (ringworm or Candida) infections, etc.

Ultraviolet and infrared lamps are very useful for treatment of a variety of diseases and have the added benefit of cosmetic use (suntan) as well as therapeutic uses (i.e., acne, eczema, arthritis, chronic infections, etc.).

Ultraviolet light can be used to diagnose certain types

of ringworm which will glow green when exposed to the ultraviolet light.

Whirlpool attachments for the tub and heating pads are very useful for both athletic types (the inevitable "sore, aching" muscles) and the arthritic patients (the "sore, aching" joints). We have also found that the "hydrotherapy" produced by the whirlpool or Jaccuzi is extremely useful for hemorrhoids (both simple and thrombosed — why get unnecessary and risky surgery?!)

The home personal computer can be brought into your "practice" for inventories, sources of medications, personal medical histories and medical records. You can also use the PC to keep track of the "payment" (chores) owed to you by your "patients" (family) for "services rendered."

Indoor exercise equipment (i.e., stationary bicycles, trampolines, treadmills, fixed or free weights, etc.) are useful physical therapy tools; they're "preventive medicine" when used to help prevent cardiovascular disease. You can afford an exceptional home "physical therapy unit" if you spend your money on equipment rather than club memberships (you will also use them more often because of the convenience — you can even watch TV while you exercise!). If you get any licensed physician to prescribe the equipment for any existing condition, insurance will pay for it; if not, the costs can be added to your tax deductible medical fees.

So you will benefit in many ways by having your own "physical therapy" department.

Now you know what "orthodox" doctors have always known about "medical toys" — why pay leasing fees for a pleasure boat out of your own pocket when "the practice" can buy the "toy" as an investment. You see, it doesn't matter that "the practice" owns the boat, the "orthodox" doctor still gets to use the boat!

TABLE 4-1. Normal Blood Pressure Chart

NORMAL BLOOD PRESSURE							
	Systolic Range			Diastolic Range			
Age	Minimum	Average	Maximum	Minimum	Average	Maximum	Pulse Pressure
15-19	105	117	129	73	77	81	40
20-24	108	120	132	75	79	83	41
25-29	109	121	133	76	80	84	41
30-34	110	122	134	77	81	85	41
35-39	110	123	135	78	82	86	41
40-44	112	125	137	79	83	87	42
45-49	115	127	139	80	84	88	43
50-54	116	129	142	81	85	89	44
55-59	118	131	144	82	86	90	45
60-64	121	134	147	83	87	91	47

Chapter 5
Medical Laboratory

"In these days when a student must be converted into a physiologist, a physicist, a chemist, a biologist, a pharmacologist and an electrician, there is no time to make a physician out of him."
— Andrew MacPhail

The "medical laboratory" is another "privilege" to which the "orthodox" doctor gets access. These laboratories do blood tests, urine tests, fecal examinations, six-hour glucose tolerance tests, pregnancy tests and check for parasites in addition to more complex functions (i.e., bacterial, viral and fungal cultures; bacterial antibiotic sensitivities; biopsy and PAP smear diagnosis, etc.). It has been a great boon to us all that American ingenuity has produced economical home test kits for almost all of the tests necessary for the "primary health care provider" (you!!!).

Allergy testing can easily be accomplished at home by two simple methods. The first is the "pulse test" which can detect allergies to foods, chemicals, cigarette smoke and pollens. The first requirement of the test is to determine what your base pulse rate is per minute. Upon awakening, double check your pulse rate, then eat or drink the suspected food, smell the suspected chemical or smoke, sniff the suspected pollen or dust then recheck your pulse rate in 15, 30 and 60 minutes. If your pulse rate goes up ten points, then you are allergic to that food or substance. You should continue to perform this test on all foods in your normal eating routine. The "pulse test" is based on the fact that when you contact an allergic substance, your heart rate (thus your pulse rate) goes up. An extreme example of this phenomena is the allergy to MSG (monosodium glutamate) or the "Chinese restaurant syndrome."

The "Chinese restaurant syndrome" is a classical food allergy to MSG. For people who are sensitive to MSG, any contact with MSG causes heart "palpitations" (skipped or irregular beats) and/or "tachycardia" (increased heart and pulse rate).

The second method for home allergy testing is the "diet diary." This technique is particularly useful in finding foods that cause allergic headaches, migraine headaches and emotional symptoms. The "diet diary" is performed by keeping a complete record of what you eat in each meal including the time at which you eat the meal. You then record any symptoms (i.e., headaches, depression, etc.) that occur in the next 12-hour period including the time of onset of symptoms.

The thyroid test is performed by taking your basal body temperature first thing in the morning by placing a thermometer in your axilla (armpit) before stirring out of bed (be sure to shake down the thermometer the night before and place it on the night stand to prevent unnecessary movement); if your basal body temperature is less than 97.8° or less, if you have chronically cold hands and feet, and if you are slow in the morning, you most likely have poor thyroid function.

"Hyper" thyroid activity from too much thyroid supplement is easily checked by holding your arm out horizontal to the floor and observing your fingers — if they are noticeably trembling then you need to cut back on your thyroid medication (another indication is your base pulse may go up five to ten points).

Urine testing is as simple as checking your car's crankcase oil — just check the "dip stick"!! Several brands of urine "dip sticks" can tell you if you have a urinary infection (bladder or kidney), blood in your urine (infection, stones, tumors, etc.), indications of blood destructive diseases, liver disease, kidney disease, diabetes (sugar) all for about $1.50 per test!! It is amazing but "orthodox" doctors normally charge you $25.00 for this test (you see, the Pentagon doesn't have the corner on the market for overpaying $25.00 for the 25 cent washer!)

Glucosticks are available for testing blood sugar (diabetics know all about this one). The test strips alone give you a gross estimate of blood sugar when compared with the color chart on the bottle. Glucosticks can be used to detect diabetes and hypoglycemia when used to perform a six-hour glucose tolerance test (six-hour GTT). The simple fasting blood sugar alone cannot detect most cases of diabetes or hypoglycemia yet the "orthodox" doctor will continue to avoid the six-hour GTT because they don't know how to use it — they also do not believe in "hypoglycemia" so it is understandable why they don't test for it.

To perform the six-hour GTT, you do a finger prick with a sterile lancet and the drop of blood is incubated on the glucostick (on the special sensitive pad) for 30 seconds and compared with the color chart on the bottle. Again, this is a gross estimate; if you wish to do a very accurate six-hour GTT, you should purchase a "glucometer." After the "fasting" blood sugar is determined (normal is 65 to 80 mg %) then you must drink a "Glucola" (a cola flavor solution containing 100 gm of glucose in a five to ten minute period. Thirty minutes after the fasting blood sugar was taken from the results (Table 5-1) to determine if you have a normal curve, a diabetic curve or a hypoglycemic curve. It is amazing, but true, that one of these tests will pay for the glucometer!

Hemoglobinometers are available to test your own hemoglobin if you have a chronic anemia. The hemoglobin level will tell you if you have enough iron in your blood. Hemoglobinometers are extremely simple to operate. A finger prick is performed and a drop of blood is placed in the instrument, an acid stick is used to burst the RBCs so the hemoglobin level can be determined by a color comparison (this procedure is similar to that used to determine the chlorine level in a pool). If you have five daughters, if you are pregnant, or if you are a serious vegetarian, this instrument will be a wise time and money saving addition to your "medical laboratory."

Home Pregnancy tests can be purchased on an as-needed basis from the local grocery store or pharmacy. The appearance of this one test has put a serious crimp in the life style of the modern "orthodox" OB/GYN.

Related to the "medical laboratory" is the ability to translate lab data from other facilities (i.e., hospitals, doctors' offices, doctors' labs, etc.) into practical and usable information for your own survival. A special series of laboratory "short-hand" is used to convey the "secret message" to the "orthodox" doctor to prevent us from helping ourselves. What follows is a basic list of the most commonly used laboratory "shorthand" and the translations. This list will allow you to understand what your "orthodox" doctor "sees" when he rubs his chin, takes off his glasses and says "hmmm," "hmmm," "I am afraid I have some bad news for you."

One caution we need to give you is that most blood values are kept in a very narrow physiological range by one or more "homeostatic" mechanisms (i.e., this is why literally thousands of people get a "clean bill of health" following a $500 physical every year and then drop dead the following week!) so you can be very ill and present a very "normal" blood test. A good example (unfortunately the "orthodox" doctor hasn't grasped this one yet!) is calcium; you can be having "spontaneous" fractures from a raging osteoporosis and your blood calcium will always be in the normal range. This fact is so definite that I often tell an audience of 1000 or more people that I would bet everything I own that they all have a "normal" blood calcium (if it were below normal, they would be having convulsions!) yet, most of them are calcium deficient.

Laboratory "Shorthand"

CBC (complete blood count) is a general term for the complete evaluation of the cellular portion of your blood including red blood cells, white blood cells and platelets. Instead of ordering each test separately, the doctor will simply ask for a CBC.

RBC (red blood cells) are specialized cells that transport oxygen as their main function in the blood, however, they also carry a variety of nutrients and waste products as they are carried through the body by the liquid portion of our blood. Anemia (the literal translation means "without blood") refers to reduced numbers of red blood cells (i.e., hemorrhage, parasites, bone marrow disease, B-12 deficiency, folic acid deficiency, or copper deficiency) or very small cells as in the case of iron deficiency. The average healthy RBC lives for 120 days so an anemia of any kind other than hemorrhage indicates a long standing problem. Normal numbers of RBCs range from 4.5 to 5.5 x 10 mm3 in males and 3.9 to 5.0 x 10 mm3 in females.

HGB (hemoglobin) is the specialized protein in the RBC that actually binds with oxygen and carbon dioxide. Increased values are seen in B-12 deficiency (because there are fewer cells) and decreased values are characteristic of iron deficiency. Cyanide and carbon monoxide tightly bind with HGB and prevent it from binding with oxygen causing a fatal "poisoning" from oxygen deprivation. Normal levels range from 14-18 gm/100 ml in males and from 12-16 gm/100 ml in females.

HCT (hematocrit) is the percentage of RBCs in relation to the fluid (serum) portion of your blood. Decreased values indicate anemia from hemorrhage, parasites, nutritional deficiencies or chronic disease process (i.e., liver disease, cancer, etc.). Normal values range from 42-52% in males and 37-47% females.

MCV (mean corpuscular volume) is a measurement of the average size of the RBC. Elevated volumes can be due to B-12 folic acid deficiency and reduced volumes are characteristic of an iron deficiency. The normal values range from 80-90 u3 in males and 79-97 u3 in females.

*MCH (mean corpuscular hemoglobin) is a measure-*ment of the weight of HGB in each RBC. The average range is 27-32 uug.

MCHC (mean corpuscular hemoglobin concentration) is the average percent of hemoglobin in each RBC relative to the total weight of the cell. The average range is 32-36%.

WBC (white blood cell) or leukocytes are the cellular portion of your immune system. In addition to floating passively in the blood stream from place to place, the

WBCs have the ability to squeeze between the cells in the blood vessel wall and attack invaders such as bacteria, viruses, parasites, cancers and foreign bodies (i.e., splinters, etc.). Viewing the WBCs reaction to food extracts under the microscope is the basis for the "cytotoxic" food allergy test.

The total WBC count is composed of five basic types of cells – determining the percentage of each type of WBC is referred to as a "deferential" and is of great value in diagnosis of infections, parasites, allergies, leukemias, appendicitis, etc. The normal range for WBC totals is 4.3 to 10.8 x 10 mm ^{3}. Deferential WBC is useful in determining many types of invasive processes in the body.

Neutrophil (segmenters or polys) are WBCs which are very active and respond quickly to invading bacteria, viruses, parasites, foreign bodies and cancer. The normal range is 40-60%. When a call for large numbers of "polys" occurs, a body throws immature "stab" or "band" neutrophils at the invader until production can be cranked up.

Monocytes (monos) are the largest of the WBCs and are increased in numbers in more chronic infections (i.e., mononucleosis, tuberculosis, etc.). When these WBCs escape into the tissue to attack foreign invaders, they are called macrophages. The normal range is 1 to 6%.

Eosinophils (Eos) are the most rapidly responding WBCs when you are having an acute (sudden) allergy reaction or parasitic infestation. The normal range is 0-2% (6-20% is a sure sign of allergies and/or parasites).

Basophils (Baso) respond to chronic intestinal allergies, eczema, asthma and sometimes with parasitic infestations. The normal range is 0-2%.

Platelets are actually fragments of larger cells (megakeriocytes) that originate in the bone marrow. Their function is to plug tears or cuts in blood vessel walls and thus prevent hemorrhage. The normal range is between 250,000 and 500,000.

SMAC-24 is a brief view through a "window" of time at 24 different serum (liquid portion of blood) components. Again, this test has limited value because the body vigorously attempts to maintain the blood levels of vitamins, minerals and enzymes even in the face of severe deficiency or illness. The classic approach is for the "orthodox" doctor to take a fasting blood sample. Few doctors can afford the expense of SMAC-24 equipment for personal use so they use the hospital "privilege" and "check you into the hospital for a few days to run some tests" or use the services of a private lab. All you really need to do is call your doctor and get him to order the lab test over the phone — this will allow you to avoid the office visit fee and the waiting room marathon. If "your" M.D. refuses to "grant" your request, check with your N.D. and/or D.C. Don't forget you are guaranteed your right of choice by the Constitution of the United States. Look in your yellow pages for the nearest N.D. and/or D.C.; if you are in one of the few states that don't have these alternative health care practitioners, get on your state congressman and state senator for a "Boston (herbal) tea party."

Glucose (fasting) is the form that blood sugar is found in your body. Elevated levels are found in diabetes ("hyper"glycemia) and low glucose value ("hypo"glycemia) is found in the 4th hour of a six-hour GTT. Blood sugar can be affected by pancreatic tumors (benign and malignant), liver disease, adrenal gland exhaustion, brain lesions and nutritional deficiencies of the trace minerals vanadium chromium. The normal range for fasting blood glucose is 65-80 mg/100 ml of blood (mg %). Elevations of the "fasting" blood sugar up to 110 mg % are considered normal by the "orthodox" medical "community," however, in reality it is a signal to get a six-hour GTT. Fasting blood sugar of 35-50 mg % is almost always a sure sign of an insulin producing pancreatic tumor or hyperinsulinemia.

Uric Acid is a barometer of protein metabolism in the liver. It is also the blood substance that accumulates to high levels in attacks of gout. The normal range is 4-8 mg % in males and 4.5-5.5 mg % in females.

Cholesterol is considered by everyone to be a barometer for risk of cardiovascular disease including arteriosclerosis and vascular thrombosis (travascular blood clots) or stroke. Elevated levels are indicative of liver disease, cardiovascular disease, diabetes, stress and low thyroid function. Low levels are characteristic of severe intestinal malabsorption and "hyper" thyroid conditions. The normal range for cholesterol is 180-200 mg % (too low can also result in life threatening problems) .

High Density Lipoproteins (HDL) are fat/protein complexes. HDL's are an integral part of the cholesterol complex and are considered desirable since they transport cholesterol to the liver for metabolism or excretion in the bile. HDLs are increased by consumption of eicosapentanoic acids (EPA — fish oils or flax seed oils). Refined sugars in your diet will lower this valuable substance to dangerous levels. The desired levels of HDL range from 30-85 mg %.

Low Density Lipoprotein (LDL) are fat/protein complexes with a high percentage of fat. The LDLs are the least desirable of the cholesterol complexes. High levels are a warning sign for increased risk of cardiovascular disease and stroke. The normal range for LDLs is 60-120 mg %.

Calcium is an essential "macro" mineral, meaning we need large amounts in our daily diet to meet our metabolic needs. Calcium is required to maintain bone density, proper neuromuscular function and blood clotting reactions. Elevated levels are rare because of the "homeostatic" mechanisms of the thyroid and parathyroid glands — when elevated calcium does occur, it signals major bone changes such as nutritional secondary hyperparathyroidism (translates to overactive parathyroid glands from chronic calcium deficiency and/or phosphorus excess) or metastasis of cancer into bone. Muscle cramps and twitches (eye twitches) are signals of calcium deficiency (although the blood calcium will be in the "normal" range). Serious life threatening convulsions from low cell levels of calcium will occur before low blood levels show up. The normal range is 9-10.8 mg %.

Phosphorus is another "macro"mineral associated with calcium, vitamin D and parathyroid function. Blood levels are again kept within very narrow physiologic limits by the parathyroid hormone. Too much phosphorus in the diet (i.e., soft drinks, meat, grains) will result in considerable calcium loss from your bones. The normal range is 3.1-4.5 mg %.

Total protein is a measure of the protein level in your serum. Low levels indicate insufficient dietary protein and/or poor digestion/absorption or liver disease. Large amounts of protein is synthesized by your liver from amino acids; this protein is released into the blood for use by any needy organ. The normal range is 6.0-6.8 mg %.

Albumin is a specialized protein produced by the liver. It helps maintain the proper fluid pressure in your blood vessels; this is why protein starved people get "edema" (i.e., fluid under the skin) or "dropsy" (i.e., fluid in the abdominal cavity). The normal range is from 3.2-5.0 mg %).

Globulin is a specialized protein produced by the liver and is primarily involved in antibody formation and antibody specificity. High levels are seen in the early stages (i.e., "acute phase") of a variety of degenerative diseases including allergies, liver disease, heart disease, arthritis, diabetes and malignancy.

A/G ratio is an abbreviation for albumin/globulin ratio. The A/G ratio is a barometer for the bodies defense system. Deviations up or down in this ratio are indications of liver disease and/or a nonspecific "flag" for chronic degenerative diseases that are exhausting the immune system. The normal range is 1.1-2.5%.

Total bilirubin is a barometer of normal metabolism of breakdown products of RBCs in the liver and spleen. Bilirubin is elevated in liver disease. Elevated bilirubin will produce jaundice of the eyes, skin and serum.

Direct bilirubin is a more specific test for liver bile

duct obstruction. Elevated levels are seen with gallstones and liver tumors. The normal range is 0-0.5 U/L.

Indirect bilirubin is a barometer of RBC destruction as well as liver function. Elevated levels are seen in anemias resulting from RBC destruction and liver/gallbladder diseases. The normal range is 0.1-1.2 U/L.

BUN (blood urea nitrogen) is a barometer of liver and kidneys ability to process the "by-products" of protein metabolism. Moderate elevations are seen in adrenal and liver disease. High elevations of BUN are a "red flag" for kidney, thyroid and anterior pituitary disease. Very low levels of BUN is typical for posterior pituitary disease. The normal range is 10-25 mg %.

Creatinine levels are a barometer of muscle metabolism and the kidneys filtering capacity. Elevated levels are "red flags" for muscle disease, kidney disease, arthritis, hyperthyroidism and diabetes. The normal range is 0.7-1.3 U/L.

BUN/Creatinine ratio is a barometer of kidney function. Elevated ratios are typical of high protein/low water diets, kidney disease and benign hypertrophy of the prostate. A decreased ratio is typical of an antidiuretic hormone insufficiency. The normal ratio is 10-35%.

Na (sodium) is an essential "macro" mineral required in our diet. Sodium is required to maintain the proper acid-base balance in our blood and tissues, the fluid pressure in our blood and tissues, the fluid pressure in our blood vessels, cells and neuromuscular function. Elevated sodium levels are characteristic of dehydration, kidney disease and adrenal gland dysfunction. Low blood levels of sodium are typical of excessive water consumption, diabetes and pituitary disorders. The normal range is 135-147 mEq/L.

K (potassium) is another one of the important "macro" minerals and is involved in maintaining proper heart rhythm, acid base balance, osmotic balance (fluid pressure) and kidney function. Elevated levels of potassium are typical of heart block, adrenal gland deficiency, and hypoventilation. Decreased potassium levels are typical of diarrhea, hyperactive adrenals, weakness, fatigue, poor posture, palpitations and irregular heartbeat and chronic kidney disease. The normal range is 3.5-4.4 mEq/L.

Cl (chloride) is involved in digestion (stomach HCl), oxygen-carrying ability of the blood, adrenal function and kidney function. Elevated levels are seen in kidney and adrenal disorders and bowel dysfunctions. Decreased levels are typical of diarrhea, infections, diabetes, reduced adrenal function. The normal range is 95-110 mEq/L.

CO_2 (carbon dioxide) is a toxic cellular waste; it is part of the acid/base balance system, initiator of involuntary lung function, kidney function and adrenal function. Elevated levels are typical of oxygen/CO_2 exchange problems (i.e., lung disease, respiratory alkalosis). Decreased levels are typical of acidosis, ketosis, etc. The normal range is 24-30 mEq/L.

LDH (lactic dehydrogenase) is an enzyme associated with carbohydrate metabolism and is widely distributed in the kidney, liver, heart, skeletal muscles and RBCs. Elevated levels are typical of injury to any of the above tissues, however, it is especially useful in monitoring heart attack, liver disease, hemolytic anemia and invasive cancers. The normal range is 60-160 u/ml.

SGOT (AST, aspartate transferase) is a transaminase enzyme associated with liver function, kidney function, heart, skeletal muscle and brain. Elevated levels are characteristic of liver and heart disease. The normal range is 0-22 u/ml.

SGPT (ALT, alanine transferase) is a transaminase enzyme associated with liver function. Elevated levels are typical of liver disease. Normal levels range from 0-22 u/ml.

Alk. Phos. (alkaline phosphatase) measures the metabolic function of bone, liver and certain tumors. Elevated levels are seen in hyperparathyroidism, bone disease, liver disease, hyperthyroidism and leukemia. Elevated levels are also seen in healing fractures and young growing bones. Normal values range from 13-40 IU/L.

GGT (gamma-glutamyl transpeptidase) is a barometer of connective tissue growth in the liver (cirrhosis), and a highly sensitive barometer of alcohol and drug abuse.

CEA (carcinoembryonic antigen) is a barometer of many malignancies (sometimes individual cancers do not affect this test). The normal levels for 97% of nonsmokers is 0-2.5 ng/ml.

PSA and ACID PHOSPHOTASE are used as a screen for prostate health — elevated levels suggest benign prostate enlargement or cancer (a biopsy may be necessary to differentiate).

OVA (eggs) of **parasites (i.e., roundworms, hookworms, and tapeworms)** and microscopic organisms (i.e., Candida albicans, bacteria, protozoa, etc.) can be found and identified in samples of feces, mucus and urine with the aid of a microscope (Fig. 5-1 &Fig. 5-2). You will need glass slides and cover slips to properly view the samples under the microscope.

Pinworms require a special diagnostic technique to identify them because of the females' habit of crawling out of the anus at night to lay eggs around the edge of the anus. A five-inch piece of clear Scotch tape is placed on the anus, sticky side toward the anus, to pick up the eggs. The tape is then placed on a slide, sticky side on the slide, and looked at through the microscope to find the eggs (Fig. 5-1).

Hair analysis is a very useful test for heavy metal toxicity (i.e., lead, mercury, arsenic, cadmium). The heavy metal levels in hair are recognized by everyone (i.e., courts, "orthodox" doctors, insurance companies, all alternative health care practitioners) as being a significant barometer of tissue levels. The nice thing about the hair analysis is that you can collect the specimen by yourself and submit it to any of the dozen of so hair analysis labs and they will give you a computerized printout that incudes an evaluation of your "macro" (i.e., calcium, phosphorus, magnesium, zinc, etc.) and trace (i.e., chromium, selenium, etc.) mineral levels.

For putting out the effort to learn the "medical laboratory" system and laboratory "shorthand" (and putting the information to proper use) you will at least add ten years to your life and at best save you from an untimely death at the hands of an "orthodox" doctor who spends more time in his investment portfolio than he does in your lab report!!!

Figure 5-1. Parasitic Ova In Fecal Samples Magnified 440x

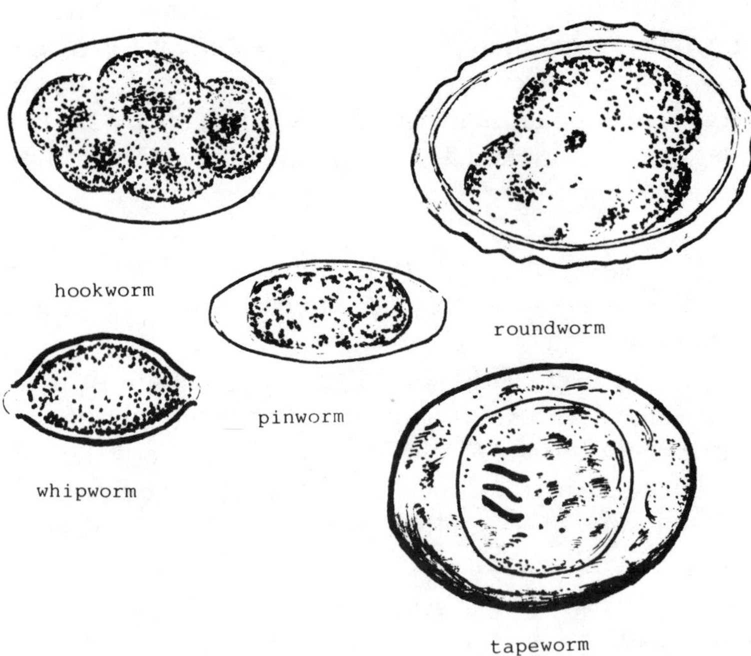

Figure 5-2. Candida, Amoeba and Bacteria Magnified 440x

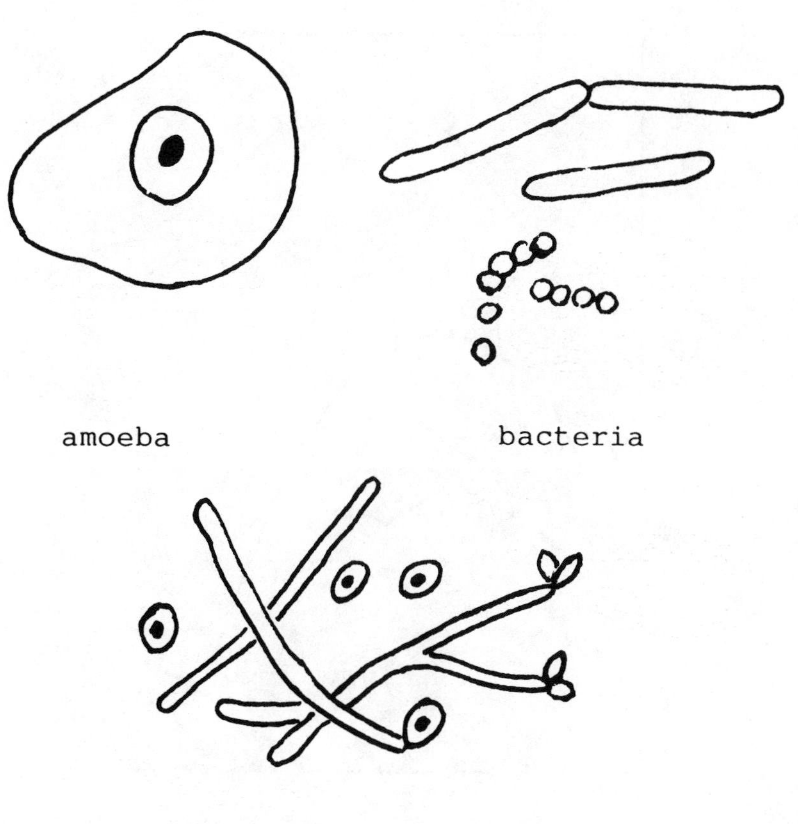

Table 5-1. Six-Hour Glucose Tolerance Test

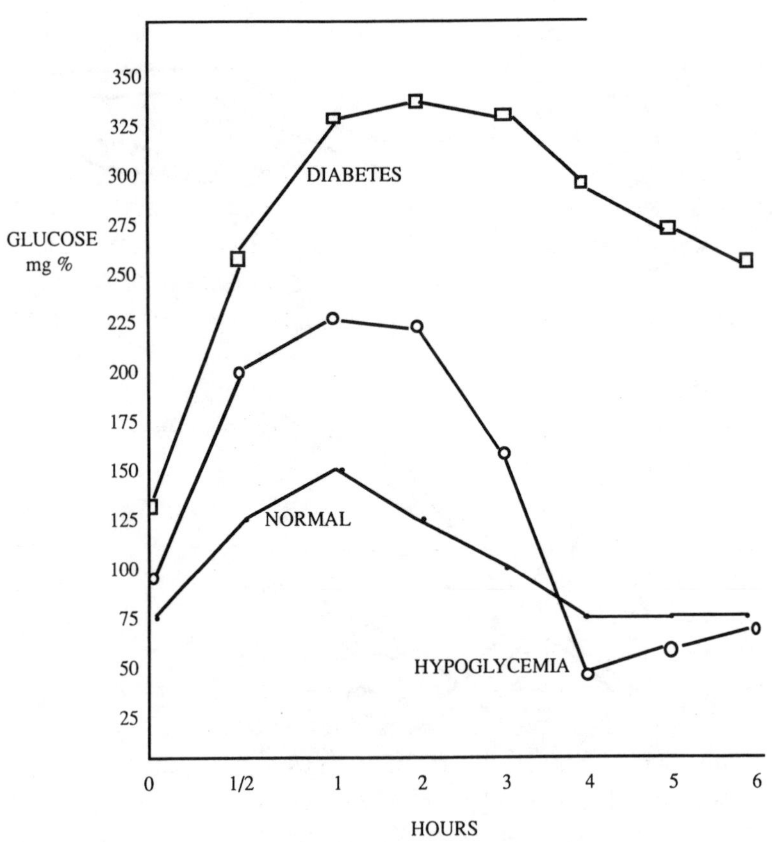

Chapter 6
Diagnosis

> *"Physicians think they are doing something for you by labeling what you have as a disease."*
>
> — Immanuel Kant

The "diagnosis" is a naming of the medical problem you have. All of the "history," "laboratory data," and "physical exam" information is used in one form or another by all of the "healing arts" as a detective uses "clues" to solve the "case." The finest example of this process is the "Sherlockian deduction" of Sherlock Holmes. Sir Arthur Conin Doyle, the creator of the "Sherlock Holmes" character, was an optometrist who had very few patients because he was shy. In his abundant spare time, he created "Holmes," basing his character on that of his pathology professor who had uncanny observational powers. His pathology professor could, by listening to their voice or footsteps deduce the patient's home country, profession or trade, diet, and medical complaint (if we only had doctors like that today!!!).

The process of "diagnosis" can be approached in two ways. The "orthodox" rut is to "rule-in" and "rule-out" based on laboratory data (no "orthodox" doctor observes anymore!!!); they go through the motions of a physical, send your blood and urine to a lab then, based on the results of these tests, they "rule-in" (consider) several possibilities which require more tests to determine which possibilities to "rule-out" and to which "specialist" to refer you! This process would be alright if "lab tests" were all revealing, however, as pointed out almost all blood and urine tests are kept in a very narrow physiological range by several body mechanisms until a life threatening crisis moves them out into a diagnostic high or low level. The batting average of this system is awful as illustrated by the statistic that only 50% of "orthodox" medical diagnosis are correct when checked at autopsy or by another physician!!!

The second and most realistic method of diagnosis is to be a highly efficient and exacting observer of the patient (who knows you better than yourself?). You must be as observant as Sherlock Holmes (remember Dr. Watson, M.D. always missed the "clues" (symptoms and signs) that were always obvious to Holmes and almost certainly missed the "solution" (diagnosis) of the case!)

What is the reason for this terrible breakdown in the competence of the "orthodox" doctor? The nurse in the doctor's office collects history, fills out forms, weighs the patients, takes BP, takes the temperature, preps you for exams, takes blood samples, gives you shots and makes your next appointment. All of these critical patient contacts are invaluable moments in which the doctor should be observing, questioning and listening to the patient's voluntary and/or subliminal comments (i.e., body language, extra comments, etc.). Unfortunately, the "orthodox" doctor has become overdependent on "labs" to "make" a "diagnosis." There are literally thousands of people who "suddenly" drop dead within 30 days after getting a "clean bill of health" from the $500 "orthodox" doctor "routine (annual) physical." Even the AMA says that the routine physicals are "cost ineffective" (this means that they rarely reveal anything of value).

I once had the opportunity to hear a lecture by the late Dr. Johnathon Leaky, the anthropologist of Oldouvi

Gorge fame, during which he said "truths are derived from facts and the more facts you have, the more reliable the truth." The same "truth" can be applied to "diagnosis" in medicine; therefore, it should not be surprising that the "orthodox" "batting average" for diagnosis and treatment is only 50%!!!

After the "orthodox" doctor's "rule-in"/"rule-out" process has been exhausted without arriving at an acceptable "diagnosis," he "refers" the patient to a "specialist" (the "orthodox" doctor's golf buddy).

If you have a heart problem, you are "referred" to a cardiologist; if you have a chronic earache, you are "referred" to an "EENT;" if you have a mysterious "lump," you are "referred" to an "oncologist" who often "refers" you to a "surgeon" or a "radiologist."

The "specialist" now puts you through his "rule-in"/"rule-out" process (this usually includes a lot of "confirming duplication" of tests because he knows from experience not to trust the original lab results as it only has a 50% chance of being correct!!!).

"Orthodox" diagnosis tends to be named after people (i.e., Swachman's Syndrome) since they are symptomatic diagnosis (i.e., depression). The most blatant offenders are the "psychiatrists." The "diseases" they "treat" are really symptoms that they try to manage (i.e., mania, depression, hysteria, paranoia, hyperactivity, etc.) rather than understanding the basic nature of the disease (i.e., PMS, hypoglycemia, food allergies or sensitivities, nutrient deficiencies, etc.).

I once had a patient from Canada who had been institutionalized for seven years for "neurosis." This woman was 32 years old, had a lovely family (including three small children) who she only saw on furloughs from the state hospital. After her original "orthodox" doctor had exhausted his "rule-in"/"rule-out" process, he "referred" her to a psychiatrist. The psychiatrist put her through the paces of his "rule-in" / "rule-out" routine; after he had exhausted all of his "orthodox" probes, he placed her in a state institution with a "diagnosis" of "depression" and exhausted his drug list trying to "stabilize" her. Since this psychiatrist had a busy practice and he got a monthly "referral check" from the institution, he sort of forgot her.

A full allergy exam and a six-hour GTT were performed on this woman with the result that she was extremely allergic to cow's milk and also was hypoglycemic. Three weeks of avoidance of cow's milk, autoimmune urine therapy and an intense therapy program for hypoglycemia and this lady was miraculously "cured" and returned to "normal" emotional health!!!

A second example was a 42 year old actor who had an "acute attack" of manic depression and self-destructive "neurosis" (he tried to stab himself to death) in London two years before we saw him. He had "depression," "paranoia," "psychosis" with "hallucinations," "catatonia" and "night terrors." After being "treated" in London with three antidepressant drugs and sleeping pills for one year, he was then "referred" to a "private" mental hospital in Spain. He remained there for one year where their "treatment" was a change from English tranquilizers to Spanish brands!

We ran a full allergy test battery and six-hour GTT on him and found that he was a severe prediabetic with a one-hour blood sugar level of 319 mg % and a "crash and burn" hypoglycemic with a low of 38 mg %; all of his "diseases" were expressed as symptoms during the test. A duplicate set of symptoms were elicited by a milk allergy. In one month's time, this patient was miraculously "cured" and happily back to work acting; his only "treatment" was avoidance of sugar and cow's milk, autoimmune urine therapy and an intensive therapy program for hypoglycemia.

The second method of "diagnosis" (and the most accurate) is to collect the facts and "rule-out" the impossible "diagnosis" (i.e., child with a cold, you automatically "rule-out" blindness, fractures, etc.) based on the facts; after awhile, the true diagnosis becomes self-evident by simple "deduction" — "It's elementary, Watson!" This method requires an acute and time consuming observational power which most "orthodox" doctors are not willing to develop.

Your diagnostic efforts will be of greatest value and accuracy if you have a "normal" baseline to refer to (i.e., BP, pulse, six-hour GTT, weight, physical inspection of remote areas (i.e., tonsils, ears, anus, prostate, vagina, cervix, etc.). Do a pulse test even if you don't think you have allergies.

When you are sick, refer to the nutrient/toxicity flow chart (Table 6-1) will give you answers to 90% of your problems. To underline this fact, one 1986 study of chronic hospital patients showed that 55% suffered from some form of overt malnutrition that "orthodox" medicine recognized (if "they" recognized it, you know it was serious!!!)

Table 6-1. Nutrient Deficiency / Toxicity Flow Chart

BIOTIN DEFICIENCY
- alopecia
- anemia
- anorexia and nausea
- depression
- fatigue
- hypercholesterolemia
- hyperglycemia (diabetes)
- insomnia
- muscle pain
- muscle weakness
- dry, greyish skin
- pale smooth tongue

CALCIUM DEFICIENCY
- arthritis
- bone spurs
- brittle fingernails
- cognitive impairment
- delusions
- depression
- eczema
- hyperactivity
- hypertension
- insomnia
- irritability
- limb numbness
- muscle cramps
- nervousness
- neuromuscular excitability
- osteomalacia
- osteoporosis
- palpitations
- paresthesia
- periodontal disease
- pica (eating lead paint)
- rickets
- retarded growth
- tetany
- tooth decay

CALCIUM TOXICITY
- anorexia
- aphasia
- ataxia
- depression
- irritability
- memory loss
- muscle weakness
- psychosis
- arrhythmias
- fat intolerance
- gastric ulcers
- growth retardation
- hypertension
- kidney disease
- liver impairment

CHROMIUM DEFICIENCY
- anxiety
- fatigue
- hypoglycemia
- diabetes
- retarded growth / short life span
- hypercholesterolemia

CHROMIUM TOXICITY
- dermatitis
- G I ulcers
- kidney dysfunction
- liver dysfunction

COPPER DEFICIENCY
- alopecia
- anemia (microcytic)

Table 6-1. Nutrient Deficiency / Toxicity Flow Chart (Continued)

aneurysm / cerebral hemorrage
criminal behavior
depression
dermatosis
diarrhea
fatigue
fragile bones / arthritis
hypercholesterolemia
otosis ("lipping" of epiphyseal plates)
respiratory disease
weakness / liver cirritosis
Swachman's syndrome

COPPER TOXICITY
depression
irritability
joint pain
muscle pain
nervousness

FOLIC ACID DEFICIENCY
anemia (megaloblastic)
anorexia
apathy
birth defects (spina bifida, hydroencephalocoele)
G I upsets/diarrhea
dyspepsia
fatigue
geographic tongue
growth retardation
headache
insomnia
memory loss
paranoia
vitaligo
weakness

ESSENTIAL FATTY ACID DEFICIENCY
acne
alopecia
arthritis
atrophy of endocrine glands
diarrhea
dry brittle hair
eczema
endocrine dysfunction
fatty degeneration of the liver
gall stones
growth retardation
immunologic dysfunction
impaired wound healing
infertility
kidney dysfunction
positive sweat test (cystic fibrosis, anorexia nervosa, etc.)
xerosis

INOSITOL DEFICIENCY
alopecia
constipation
eczema
hypercholesterolemia

IODINE DEFICIENCY
goiter
fatigue
hypothyroidism
low basal body temperature
weight gain

Table 6-1. Nutrient Deficiency / Toxicity Flow Chart (Continued)

IRON DEFICIENCY
- anemia (microcytic)
- angular stomatitis
- anorexia
- brittle nails
- confusion
- constipation
- depression
- dizziness
- dysphagia
- fatigue
- fragile bones
- G I upset
- growth retardation
- headaches
- ice eating (pica)
- irritability
- palpitations

IRON TOXICITY
- anorexia
- dizziness
- fatigue
- headaches

MAGNESIUM DEFICIENCY
- anxiety/confusion/ irritability/restlessness
- birth defects
- depression
- hyperactivity/sonophobia
- hypotension
- hypothermia
- insomnia
- muscle pain/muscle tremors/ muscle weakness
- nervousness/neuromuscular irritability
- SIDS
- seizures
- tachycardia/palpitations

MANGANESE DEFICIENCY
- ataxia
- atherosclerosis
- dizziness
- hearing loss
- hypercholesterolemia
- hypoglycemia
- muscle therapy
- pancreatic atrophy
- tinnitus

MANGANESE TOXICITY
- anorexia
- impaired judgement
- Parkinsonism
- memory loss

NIACIN DEFICIENCY
- anorexia & nausea
- canker sores
- confusion
- depression
- dermatitis
  - localized scaly, dark pigmented dermatitis
- diarrhea
- crying jags, emotional
- fatigue
- halitosis (bad breath)
- headache
- dyspepsia
- insomnia
- irritability

Table 6-1. Nutrient Deficiency / Toxicity Flow Chart (Continued)

limb pains
memory loss
muscular weakness
skin eruptions/eczema

NIACIN TOXICITY
niacin "flush"
liver impairment

PANTOTHENIC ACID (B-5) DEFICIENCY
abdominal pain
alopecia
burning feet
coordination impairment
depression
eczema
faintness
fatigue
hypotension
infections
insomnia
muscle spasms
nausea & vomiting
nervousness
tachycardia
weakness

PARA AMINOBENZOIC ACID (PABA) DEFICIENCY
constipation
depression/headache/irritability
G I disorders
fatigue
graying hair

PHOSPHORUS DEFICIENCY
anorexia
anxiety
apprehension
bone pain
dyspnea
fatigue
irritability
numbness
paresthesias
pica
tremulousness
weakness
weight loss

PHOSPHORUS TOXICITY
calcium malabsorption
loose teeth
osteoporosis / arthritis
secondary hyperparathyroidism
tooth loss
weight loss

POTASSIUM DEFICIENCY
acne
arrhythmia
cognitive impairment
constipation
depression
ECG changes
edema
fatigue
glucose intolerance
growth retardation
hypercholesterolemia
hyperreflexia
hypotension

Table 6-1. Nutrient Deficiency / Toxicity Flow Chart (Continued)

- insomnia
- muscle weakness
- nervousness
- palpitations
- polydipsia
- proteinuria
- respiratory distress
- "salt"" retention
- tachycardia (rapid heart rate)
- xerosis

POTASSIUM TOXICITY

- cardiac arrest
- cognitive impairment
- dysarthria
- dysphasia
- weakness

PYRIDOXINE (B-6) DEFICIENCY

- acne
- alopecia
- anemia
- anorexia & nausea
- arthritis
- cheilosis
- conjunctivitis
- depression
- dizziness
- facial oiliness
- fatigue
- geographic tongue
- impaired wound healing
- irritability
- nervousness
- neurologic symptoms
- seizures
- stomatitis
- stunted growth
- weakness

PYRIDOXINE TOXICITY

- "electric shock" sensations
- paresthesia

RIBOFLAVIN (B-2) DEFICIENCY

- alopecia
- blurred vision
- cataracts
- cheilosis
- depression
- dermatitis (drying, greasy, scaling)
- dizziness
- eyes (itching, burning, red)
- geographic tongue
- growth retardation
- pancreatic atrophy & fibrosis
- photophobia

SELENIUM DEFICIENCY

- cataracts
- cancer risk
- cystic fibrosis
- growth retardation
- "heart attack"
- impaired immunity
- Keshan Disease (myocardial fibrosis)
- muscular dystrophy
- pancreatic atrophy & fibrosis (cystic fibrosis)
- liver cirrhosis
- sterility in males

Table 6-1. Nutrient Deficiency / Toxicity Flow Chart (Continued)

SELENIUM TOXICITY
- alopecia
- arthritis
- brittle nails
- garlic breath
- metallic taste
- kidney dysfunction
- liver dysfunction

SODIUM DEFICIENCY
- abdominal cramps
- anorexia
- ataxia
- confusion
- crying jags
- depression
- dermatosis
- dizziness
- fatigue
- flatulence
- hallucinations
- headaches
- hypotension
- illusions
- infections
- lethargy
- memory loss
- muscular weakness
- nausea & vomiting
- seizures
- taste loss
- weight loss

SODIUM TOXICITY
- anorexia
- cognitive dysfunction
- congestive heart failure
- edema (especially low protein diets)
- hyperactivity
- hypertension
- hypertonia
- irritability
- polydipsia
- polyuria
- renal failure
- seizures
- tremors
- weight gain

VITAMIN B-1 DEFICIENCY
- anorexia
- brain atrophy (senility)
- confusion
- constipation
- coordination impairment
- depression
- dyspnea (labored breathing)
- G I upset
- edema
- fatigue
- irritability
- memory loss
- muscle atrophy
- nervousness
- numbness hands and feet
- pain hypersensitivity
- palpitations
- sonophobia
- weakness

VITAMIN B-12 DEFICIENCY
- achlorhydria
- anemia
- birth defects
- constipation

Table 6-1. Nutrient Deficiency / Toxicity Flow Chart (Continued)

- depression
- dizziness
- dyspnea (labored breathing)
- fatigue
- G I upset
- geographic tongue
- headache
- irritability
- moodiness
- numbness
- palpitations
- psychosis
- spinal cord degeneration

VITAMIN A DEFICIENCY

- acne
- anosmia (loss of smell)
- birth defects
- dry hair/alopecia
- fatigue
- growth retardation
- hyperkeratosis
- infections
- infertility
- insomnia
- night blindness
- weight loss
- xerophthalmia
- xerosis

VITAMIN A TOXICITY

- abdominal pain
- alopecia
- amenorrhea
- cheilosis
- G I upset
- hepatomegaly
- hydrocephalus
- irritability
- joint pain
- nausea & vomiting
- pruritis
- splenomegaly
- weight loss

VITAMIN C DEFICIENCY

- bleeding gums/loose teeth
- depression/malaise/tiredness
- easy bruising
- impaired would healing
- irritability
- joint pain

VITAMIN D DEFICIENCY

- burning in mouth
- burning in throat
- diarrhea
- insomnia
- myopia
- nervousness
- osteomalacia
- rickets

VITAMIN D TOXICITY

- angiotoxicity (calcification)
- arteriosclerosis (angiotoxicity)
- liver dysfunction
- "malignant" calcification

VITAMIN E DEFICIENCY

- alopecia
- areflexia
- dermatitis
- gait disturbances

Table 6-1. Nutrient Deficiency / Toxicity Flow Chart (Continued)

infertility
malabsorption
muscular dystrophy
ophthalmoplegia
proprioception problems
RBC fragility
vibratory sense dysfunction

VITAMIN K DEFICIENCY
poor clotting time
osteoporosis

VANADIUM DEFICIENCY
diabetes
hypoglycemia

ZINC DEFICIENCY
acne
alopecia
anorexia
apathy
birth defects
brittle nails
depression
eczema
fatigue
growth retardation
hypercholesterolemia
hypogeusia (loss of sensation of taste)
impaired wound healing
impotence
infertility
irritability
lethargy
malabsorption
memory loss
paranoia
sexual immaturity
sterility
white spots on nails

Chapter 7
Healing Arts

"The secret of caring for the patient is caring for the patient."
— Sir William Osler

"Orthodox" western doctors would have us believe that "theirs is the only medical system of any value." We are taking the "liberty" to briefly outline several healing arts that are currently being used by 2/3 of the peoples of the earth, some of which have been around for 10,000 years (the "orthodox" American system of medicine has only been around since the 1914 Flexner Report — this is typical of their arrogance!)

ACUPUNCTURE is an ancient therapy based on the premise that there are channels of energy (meridians) that flow through the body with specific points that represent organs and organ systems. Acupuncture involves the placement of very fine needles into the specific points to rechannel energy so as to treat an organ, organ system or produce analgesia.

Acupuncture is an ancient Chinese healing art dating from before 3500 BC. It was originally observed that warriors pierced by arrows frequently reported relief from chronic diseases; it was these battlefield observations that led to the development of acupuncture meridians and points.

The first "official" text written on acupuncture was produced by the Yellow Emperor (Hangdi Neiging

Suwen) in 200 BC.

The Chinese list over one thousand "points" for diagnosis and treatment. Some of these "points" are recognized by Western practitioners as "referred pain" locations. These "points" are found on twelve meridians or channels. The courses of the meridians are not uniform and unique patterns and "points" must be memorized or taken from models or charts.

The Chinese call the "life force" or "spirit" Qi (pronounced Chi) which flows through the meridians. A blockage or misdirection of the Qi flow results in disease. The reestablishment of the blocked flow of energy is the goal of acupuncture.

The Chinese acupuncture system recognizes physiological circadian rhythms and interorgan relationships; it expresses them in three basic sets of parameters:

1) Yin and Yang
2) Five Main Elements
3) Time of treatment during the 24-hour clock and annual calendar

Modern needles are made of silver alloys or stainless steel. Early versions of needles were made of stone, iron, copper, bronze, ivory, etc. The needle can be inserted into the patient using more than 50 different techniques, however, seven basic factors determine the efficiency of the needle:

1) caliber of the needle
2) twirling or vibrating
3) depth of penetration
4) sharpness
5) amount of time of treatment
6) number of follow-up treatments

7) heat (moxibustion)

Any treatable and curable disease of altered physiology can be cured by acupuncture; acupuncture is also an excellent method for producing analgesia (pain relief) and/or anesthesia (pain relief with unconsciousness).

Conditions and diseases not to be treated by acupuncture:

1) infections
2) parasites
3) cardiovascular disease
4) cancer
5) kidney disease
6) diabetes, hypoglycemia, thyroid disease
7) pregnancy (can be used for analgesia during labor)
8) vaginal discharges
9) prostate disease
10) otitis media (middle ear problems)
11) emphysema
12) eye disease
13) fractures
14) emergency surgical problems (appendicitis)
15) transected nerves and blood vessels

Chinese measurements are used to locate acupuncture meridians and points. The basic unit is a Cun, which is approximately the width of the widest part of the patients thumb. A fen is 1/10 of a Cun.

Accurate placement of the needle will produce a sensation or energization called "te-chi." The depth of the needle insertion is five fen (1/2 inch, or just below the skin). The needles are left in place for 20-30 minutes then removed. If a lot of treatment energy is indicated, the needles may be twirled or heated with "moxa" after insertion.

Needles should be sterilized between use by heating in an autoclave (medical sterilizer) or up to 350°F in the oven for 30 minutes. The beginner acupuncturist should wear sterile rubber gloves to prevent contamination of the needles.

Anesthesia and analgesia produced by acupuncture is very safe and doesn't need a prescription from the "orthodox" doctor! The obstetrical and surgical patient is aware of what's happening but doesn't perceive pain. Postsurgical pain is easily controlled with acupuncture. The induction of analgesia takes about 20-30 minutes; it takes from one to ten needles to produce satisfactory analgesia (beginners need ten):

TREATMENT AREA	MERIDIAN POINTS INDUCE ANALGESIA
ears	Co 4, Me 3, Me 17
eyes	Co 4, St2
esophagus	Co 4, Va 6
nose	Co 4, Co 20, St2
upper teeth	Co 4, St6, St7, St44
lower teeth	Co 4, St5, St6
throat	Co 4, St6, St44
urethra	St36, Sp6, Sx4, Br 2
uterus	St36, Sp6, Li 3, Br 4

NORMAL CHILDBIRTH AND LABOR POINTS

meridian points Co 4, Va 6, Sp6, Sp9, Li 3, Li 6, St36, St44

The best meridian charts and point locations are found in the book, Acupuncture for Americans; however, we have provided you with several basic charts to get you started (Fig. 7-1). Needles and complete charts are available through Chinese herbal shops and some herbal distributors.

Acupressure and reflexology are variations of acupuncture that were derived by the orientals. These techniques employ "points" or zones on the feet (Fig. 7-2) and body meridians to correct flow of energy to help eliminate disease.

For those too conservative to use needles (especially in the early stages of "pre-med" training), you may choose to use electroacupuncture (i.e., penlight sized "acu-spark") or the larger Vol machines for meridian diagnosis as well as electro-acupuncture therapy. The advantage of the Vol machine is that it has an indicator gauge as well as an audio signal to let you know that you are precisely on a "point!"

AROMATHERAPY is a combination of body and face massages using essential aromatic oils extracted from plants. It is practiced as one form of herbal medicine and/or beauty therapy. The "essence" of the plant source can be extracted from various parts of the plant:

ROOTS	FLOWERS	LEAVES
calamus	lavender	rosemary
BARK	RESIN	
sandalwood	myrrh	

The oils function as pesticides, fungicides, bactericides, and hormonelike substances in plants. These oils are excellent for treating scars, acne and stretch marks.

BIRTH CONTROL	Mexican yam
TESTOSTERONE	Sarsaparilla
INTESTINAL ANTISPASMODIC	peppermint, cardamon
REDUCE BLOOD PRESSURE	calamus
EXPECTORANT	lemon oil
ESTROGENS	hope, anise seed, fennel

AYURVEDIC MEDICINE is thought to be the most ancient of all medical arts. Ayurvedic medicine literally translates to "life sciences." Ayur = life, veda = science is recorded in the Arthavara veda 1200 BC. The "Sambuta," or encyclopedia of medicines, was written in 500 BC. Eighty to ninety percent of the people in India are treated with Ayurvedic medicine. It is generally thought that the western form of medicine comes from the Greeks – but the Greeks learned it from the East Indians. Pythagoras, one of Hippocrates' early teachers, obtained his whole system from India.

According to Ayurvedic medicine, at the level of the individual mind, there are three types of activity:

Rojas	active creating energy
Tamas	passive resisting or destroying energy
Satva	unifying, preserving energy

Pitta	active energy of heat
Kapha	element of phlegm (cold)
Vaya	element of air

All of the above forces are modified by the spiritual, mental and physical aspects of the patient.

The human and the universe are composed of five elements or Bhutas (which appear to be the origins of the four Greek humors:

1) Ether	sound
2) Air	light/touch
3) Fire	hot/sight
4) Water	wet/taste
5) Earth	heavy/smell

Ayurveda expects the patient to take part in his own cure. According to Ayurveda, the human body is made up of seven tissues or Dhatus; if the Dhatus are in balance, the individual is heathy. Food after digestion feeds the Dhatus; any imbalance in food creates disease in the Dhatus. Ayurvedic medicine puts great emphasis on "wrong food" as a cause of disease although it does recognize that physical activity, sleep, sexual habits, climate, emotional status, surrounds, age and gender all influence disease. Ayurvedic medicine doesn't arrive at a "diagnosis" by western standards but treats "imbalances." The ayurvedic pharmacopeia of drugs is very large having collected several thousands of compounds over a period of thousands of years. The drugs are prepared as jellies, tinctures, powders, pills or oils. Refined minerals, metals and precious stones are also used in treatments.

"Mantras" (prayer-like sayings), yogic breathing techniques and medical "ceremonies" are employed in the ayurvedic treatment programs. It is thought that homeopathy, color therapy and radiesthesia are derived from ayurvedic medicine.

Bach Remedies (Bach Flower Remedies) were conceived by Edward Bach (1880-1936). Bach started his career as a bacteriologist in the University College Hospital in London and as the pathologist and bacteriologist to the London Homeopathic Hospital. In 1926, he published a book, Chronic Diseases: A Working Hypothesis; in 1933, he wrote Heal Thy Self, the Twelve Healers. Initially, Bach collected sunwarmed dew on flowers; he eventually expanded his "remedies" to a homeopathic — like water preparation of flowers. Traditionally the patient takes four (4) drops of the diluted "remedy" four times per day. Bach's remedies were "designed" to "cure" emotional imbalances rather than physical disease.

Biochemics (Schuessler Cell Salts) is a system of medical therapy devised in the last century by a physician and chemist, Dr. Wilhelm Heinrich Schuessler. He based his "science" on the analysis of the ashes of cremated human bodies. In these ashes Schuessler found twelve (12) "salts" (minerals) basic and essential to human health. Dr. Schuessler was heavily influenced by the great German chemist, Dr. Liebig (the human body is made up of "cells" composed of organic material, water and "salts." In recent times, an additional 30 trace elements have been recognized and added to the original twelve "cell salts." Schuessler classically used homeopathic doses of the cell salts in treating his patients.

Chiropractic is a physical form of medicine that heals without the use of drugs or surgery. Chiropractic philosophy believes that many diseases, especially physical

FIGURE 7-1. Acupuncture Chart of Head and Ear Points

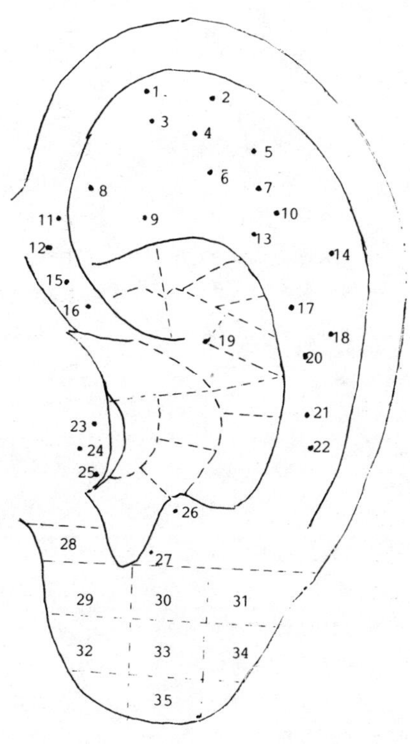

1. Toes
2. Fingers
3. Ankle
4. Shemen
5. Knee
6. Buttocks
7. Gall Bladder
8. Uterus
9. Hip
10. Abdomen
11. Sympathy
12. Genitalia
13. Lumbar
14. Elbow
15. Urethra
16. Rectum
17. Breast
18. Shoulder
19. Diaphragm
20. Thoracic
21. Neck
22. Brain
23. Pharynx
24. External Nose
25. Internal Nose
26. Gonads
27. Eye II
28. Eye I
29. Lower Teeth
30. Forehead
31. Middle Ear
32. Upper Teeth
33. Eye
34. Inner Ear
35. Tonsil

FIGURE 7-1. Acupuncture Chart of Head and Ear Points

(Continued)

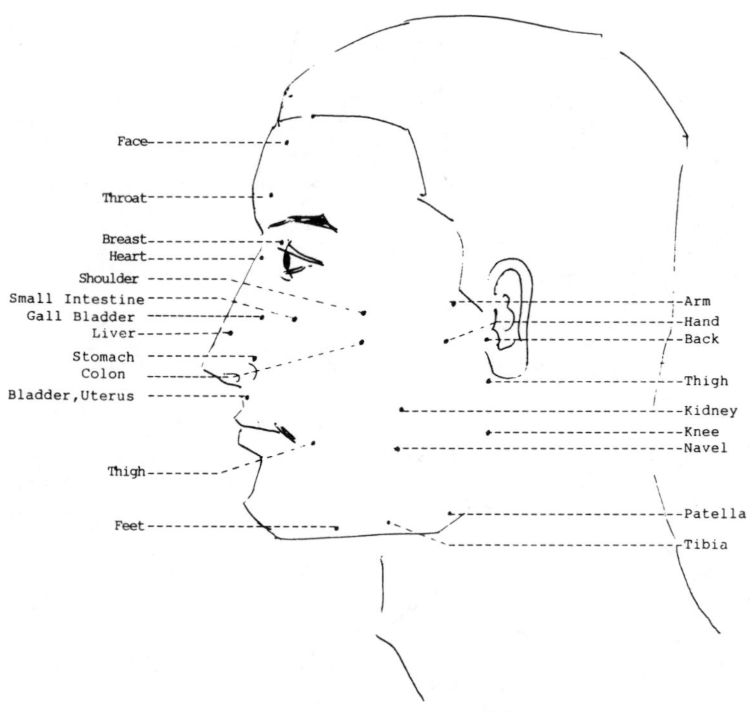

FIGURE 7-1. Foot Acupuncture Points and Reflexology Zones

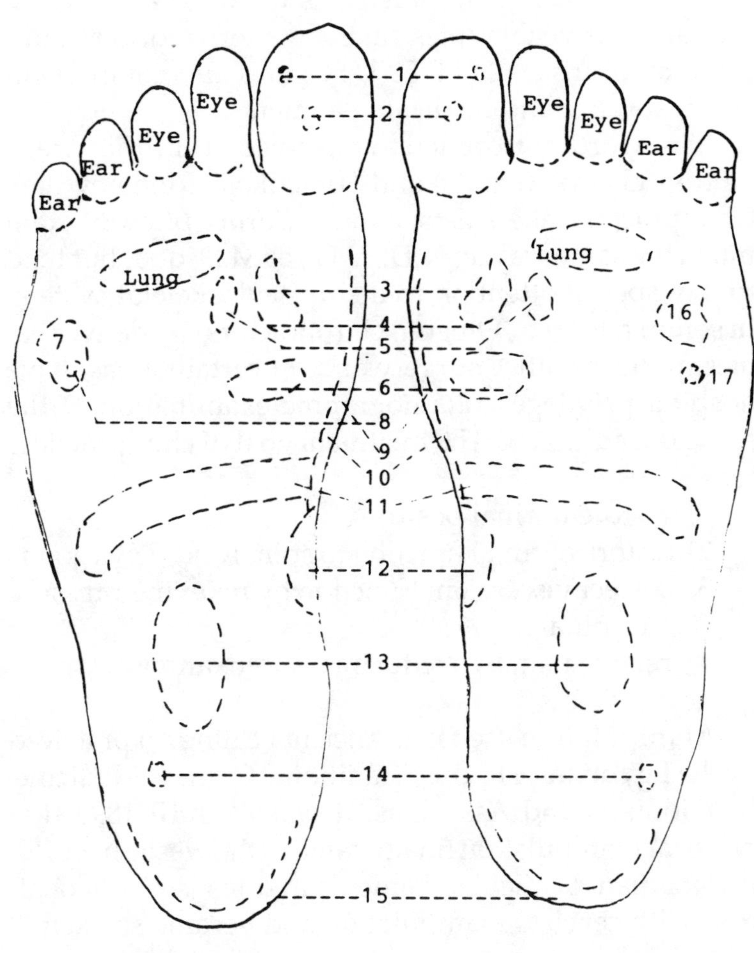

1. Scalp
2. Pituitary
3. Thyroid
4. Parathyroid
5. Thymus
6. Stomach
7. Liver
8. Gallbladder
9. Spinal Column
10. Waist
11. Large Intestine
12. Urinary Bladder
13. Small Intestine
14. Sciatic Nerve
15. Hemorrhoid
16. Heart
17. Spleen

discomfort and many visceral malfunctions are caused by "subluxations" of vertebral joints pressing on spinal nerves. Today "chiropractic" is the most accepted of the "alternative therapies" in the western world as indicated by licensure in all 50 U.S. states and comprehensive insurance and medicare payments.

The word chiropractic is derived from the Greek words "cheiro" (hands) and "practikos" (done by the). Chiropractors take a history and perform a physical exam much the same way an N.D., D.O., or M.D. does but tend to pay special attention to the musculoskeletal system. In some states (i.e., Oregon) chiropractors can deliver babies, perform office surgery and, in certain areas, have hospital privileges. Radiographic examination of the spine is traditional. The treatment goal of chiropractic is to:

1) restore normal posture
2) restore optimal function to spinal and pelvic joints
3) correct visceral malfunction by relieving pressure on spinal nerves
4) relieve pain by "reducing" subluxations

Manipulation itself is an ancient healing art practiced by the Egyptians, Hindus, Traditional Chinese Medicine, Babylonians and Assyrians. It wasn't until 1895 that physical manipulation finally came to the western world. A Canadian, Daniel D. Palmer, cured his janitor's deafness with cervical manipulation and became so excited with this "new" therapy that he abandoned his interest in mesmerism (hypnotism) and magnetic healing. Palmer soon founded the Palmer Infirmary and Chiropractic Institute in Iowa.

The chiropractic profession has been at odds with the "orthodox" medical profession since its inception. In 1987, the chiropractors finally won a landmark case against the AMA for conspiracy to break the U.S. antitrust laws. The AMA is now blocked from openly trying to destroy chiropractic (this ruling has had the effect of keeping the AMA from attacking other healing arts (i.e., naturopathic physicians, etc.). The nice thing about chiropractic is that certain basic treatments are easily learned and it can be employed in the home.

Color therapy is the use of colored lights or panels to create a positive healing effect. Color therapy was originally recorded in the Greek Healing Temples of light and color at Heliopolis, Egypt. Color healing is also used in ayurvedic and traditional Chinese medicine; the gem therapy of ayurvedic medicine is a close parallel in theory and methodology.

The color blue appears to be the universally favored color, followed by red. It is well documented that our response to color is emotional; our response to shape is intellectual. It is also agreed upon that certain forms of sound and light are therapeutic — color therapy is considered by many to be another form of light therapy:

1) Blue reduces BP, alleviates teething, boils, fever, inflammation, dysentery, colic, jaundice and heals cuts and burns

2) Red alleviates "hypo"tension and certain forms of paralysis

3) Yellow/Violet alleviates anxiety and arthritis

4) Orange alleviates gallstones and kidney stones

5) Yellow - diabetes and constipation

6) Green - ulcers, colds, flu, breast cancer

Color therapy techniques include:

1) Kilner screen — a diagnostic tool. Consists of two (2) plates of glass with a solution of diocene (indigo/violet solution); the color therapist views the patient through the screen to determine which colors are needed

2) Tissue colors — a diagnostic tool. The color therapist observes the color of the sclera (white of the eye), nails, urine and stool

3) Solar-chrome salt bags — a therapy tool. Massage patient with colored salt in a cheesecloth sack. These bags are "charged" by exposure to the sun or sunlamps for one hour prior to the massage.

4) Food colors — a therapy tool. Select food colors that will treat the patient. Colored food groups contain specific "chemicals" (vitamins and minerals) needed by the patient.

5) Rainbow healing — a therapy tool. Water is placed in colored glasses and exposed to sunlight. The water takes on the healing qualities of the specific color and it is passed onto the patient who drinks it.

6) Color breathing — a therapy tool. A style of retiring and awakening-meditation.

Laying-on-of-hands (spiritual and faith healers) — the use of a human to mediate healing. "Healers" were recorded in ancient China, Egypt and in various forms today in Christianity. A spiritual healer works on the premise that whatever one believes can be made to happen by belief in God. Spiritual healing works through contact with the "world of spirits," mediums and psychic phenomena. "Positive thinking" is practiced by Christians and alternative physicians alike. Robert Schuller considers positive thinking to be a form of prayer. Twenty to sixty percent of patients will recover with placebos if positive thought is induced.

Christian Scientists are a sect of orthodox Christians founded in 1879 by Mary Baker Eddy (Church of Christ, Scientists) who believed that "healing is proof of God's love for man." Statistically Christian Scientists live longer than any group of western people and, as a result, have special lower insurance premiums.

It is of interest that Kirlian photography shows a significant increase in the healer's hand "aura" during "laying-on-of-hands." A new-age concept of "laying-on-of-hands" is "therapeutic touch" which is practiced by nurses and massage therapists on patients with poor circulation and debilitating diseases.

Herbal medicine is an ancient system of medicine that uses plants to prevent and cure disease. Traditional Chinese medicine, ayurvedic medicine, American Indian medicine, American folk medicine, Eclectic medicine and naturopathic medicine all have strong roots in herbal medicine.

The Chinese had large complex pharmacopeias in 3000 B.C. and the Persians are said to have used plants medicinally as long ago as 6,000 years! An Assyrian, King Asurbipal, had a list of 250 plant drugs in 2500 B.C. In 1653, Nicholas Culpeper published the "Complete Herbal." Even today, more than thirty percent of today's "orthodox" pharmaceuticals are derived from herbal compounds (i.e., digitalis, foxglove, and vincristine — a CA therapy from the Madagascar periwinkle). The seventeenth century produced the "Doctrine of Signatures" which puts forth the theory that certain plants and plant parts looked like various human organs as a "God-given clue" to what medicinal value each had.

Herbal medicines have the advantage of safety (there are exceptions!!!) and thousands of years of experience. Currently herbal preparations are easy to procure in tablet, capsule, tea bag and fluid (i.e., extracts and elixirs) preparations. Herbs are also easy to cultivate at home in significant quantities making them very attractive to retired people on fixed incomes and young families with lots of expenses but small incomes.

Homeopathy is a widely practiced medical art that has two basic principles:

1) "let like be cured by like"

2) principle of "minimum dose"

Agents (herbs, chemicals, etc.) produce certain symptoms in normal healthy humans ("proved") — these agents are then used to cure diseases that produce the "proved" symptoms.

Dr. Samuel Hahnemann, a physician from Leipzig, Germany, "proved" that Cinchona bark (a malaria cure of the day) gave malaria symptoms to healthy people. Hahnemann went on to "prove" hundreds of medications and substances. He also found that very frequently the more dilute the preparation, the more dramatic the clinical effect (Table 7-1). This observation has been the center of controversy since Hahnemann's time. It is of interest that in 1988 a significant article was published in Nature magazine that supports Hahnemann's observations!!!

There are two basic forms of homeopathic remedies - the dilutions are known as "potencies" (Table 7-2):

1) solid remedies are ground up with lactose (milk sugar) by a process known as "trituration." The "active" substance is diluted 10 fold with the lactose.

2) Liquid remedies are mixed with alcohol and shaken, a process known as "succussion" — again liquid remedies are diluted ten fold. The strength or "potency" of the remedy is expressed as 1C, 2C, 3C, etc. as each successive 100 fold dilution and "succussion" is made.

English homeopathic remedies are labeled 1X, 2X, and 3X while European designations 1D, 2D, and 3D are used to indicate decimal or ten fold dilutions. At 12C or 1024, there may be one molecule or none of the original substance (Avogadro's Law) yet the "remedy" will have a homeopathic medical effect!!!

Hydrotherapy began in Roman times and is widely used today by all forms of healing arts including "orthodox" medicine. The medicinal baths take many forms from "sitz" baths for hemorrhoids, whirlpool for muscle injuries to mineral baths for arthritis. Many times insurance companies will pay for some form of hydrotherapy if it is prescribed by a licensed physician of any healing art.

Hydrotherapy takes many forms including:

1) <u>cold bath</u> – reduces swelling

2) <u>hot bath</u> – relieves soreness and improves circulation for chronic diseases and injuries

3) <u>mineral bath</u> – for chronic disease - i.e., arthritis

4) <u>steam bath</u> – detox heavy metals

5) sitz bath – hemorrhoids

6) epsom salt bath – produces sweating, relieves edema and soreness and will clean infected wounds

7) water fast – detoxification of food allergies and can be used as a prelude to diagnosing food allergies

8) colonic irrigation - constipation, detoxify patients being treated for any chronic disease or liver ailment (infectious hepatitis would be an exception)

9) knipping - walking or jogging in knee-deep water of a lake or ocean for stimulating circulation and immune system

TABLE 7-1. Homeopathic Remedy Potencies and Terminology

DILUTION	CONCENTRATION		DECIMAL SCALE	CENTESIMAL
1/10	10%	10(-1)	D1 or 1x	1C
1/100	1%	10(-2)	D2 or 2x	
1/1,000	0.1%	10(-3)	D3 or 3x	
1/10,000	0.01%	10(-4)	D4 or 4x	2C
1/100,000	0.001%	10(-5)	D5 or 5x	
1/1,000,000	0.0001%	10(-6)	D6 or 6x	3C
1/1,000,000,000,000	AVOGADRO'S LAW	10(-12)	D12 or 12x	6C

TABLE 7-2. Abbreviated Repertory

REPERTORY - "Cook Book" collection of symptoms and remedies. Find description of patients illness by symptoms and pick out correct remedy.

MATERIA MEDICA - List of homeopathic remedies and methods of preparation.

MOTHER TINCTURE - The original concentrated homeopathic remedy used as a storage form to conserve space.

POLYCRESTS - Remedies that give a wide range of symptoms in the provers (i.e., Sulphur, Pulsatilla, Lycopodium, Phosphorus, etc.)

ACONITE - Sudden chill, fever, thirst, roar in ears, sleepiness, sneezing, acutely inflamed throat. Croup, dry cough, spasmodic cough. Restless, anxious, frightened. Sudden onset, worse at night.

ALLIUM CEPA - Cold with intense coryza, feels thick in head, worse in warm room plus sneezing, eyes red with profuse bland lacrimation, watering eyes and nose, upper lip red and sore, better in open air.

ARSENICUM ALBUM - Pouring water from nose, excoriating upper lip. Sneezing from focal irritation, always catching cold from changes in weather, begins in nose and travels to chest. Chilly, worse in draughts (HEPAR), freezing, hugs fire (NUX). Chilly with burning, better from heat, restless, anxious, ice cold blood through vessels. Asthmatic type of cough, dry hacking with no expectoration. Thirst for constant sips of cold water.

BELLADONNA - Sudden chill and violent onset of bronchitis. Begins with sore, red shiny throat. Intense mental excitement. Pain very acute, worse with slightest movement, violent pulsating headache, flushed intense burning heat, dilated pupils, dry red tongue with thirst.

BRYONIA - Cold going on to chest, hoarse and sore at back of throat. Goes on to cough which shakes patient to bits and is very painful over the top of the chest. Holds chest on coughing and

TABLE 7-2. Abbreviated Repertory (Continued)

head because of headache. Short hacking dry cough, better lying on affected side, much worse from motion. Very thirsty for long, cold drinks, very hot, wants to be left alone, looks drugged and bluish. Cough of measles.

GELSIMIUM - Colds which come on days after exposure in warm, moist relaxing weather. History of feeling chilled after being too hot several days before. Doesn't notice windows open. Chilliness and shivers up and down back in spite of being hot and sticky. Acute fluid coryza and sneezing. Although hot, has cold extremities and is sitting by fire particularly with flu. Aching, and heavy all over with soreness of muscles. May get tickley cough or more croupy kind of cough. Headache severe in flu over head and eyes. Mild dislike of disturbance. Headache better with passing of urine. If excited will have sleepless night. Thirstless nearly always.

HEPAR SULPH - Comes on in cold dry weather, after with a sticking sensation like a splinter in the throat. Paroxysms of dry, teasing, painful cough with very sore chest and throat. Very hot but can't, or won't, move or be uncovered without feeling chilly. Sweats profusely but lies covered up to chin. No relief from sweat. Worse breathing cold air, worse putting hand out of covers. Suffocating croupy cough. Very irritable and hypersensitive. Apt to quarrel with own shadow particularly in flu and chest conditions.

ARNICA - For any injury or bruising. Falls, fractures before and after operations, where there is a history of old injury, particularly if never well since, or if left with chronic after effects.

LACHESIS - Very hot remedy, bluish appearance, left-sided remedy. All symptoms worse from heat, much worse from tight clothing or tight collar, collar must be loosened. Much worse after sleep, wakes feeling dead.
Better immediately after menstrual period onset. Menopausal remedy; very loquacious and darts from subject to subject. Very jealous and/or suspicious.

TABLE 7-2. Abbreviated Repertory (Continued)

CONSTITUTIONAL REMEDIES

TERENTULA - Mental excitement, hysteria, hallucinations. Rage, fury.

ARSINICUM ALBUM - Oversensitive, smell, touch, hair combed, anxiety, and an anxious expression

NITRIC ACID - Sensitive to touch and upset beyond reason by pain.

HEPAR SULPHURIS - Marked skin hyperaesthesia to touch, draught, personal atmosphere. Easily upset, flies into temper rage.

NUX VOMICA - Cutaneous sensitivities to cold, touch, noise, being interfered with, nerves on edge, startled if touched suddenly.

GENTIANA LUTEA - Ravenous hunger; diminished appetite

JASMINUM OFFICINALE - Comatose, vomiting, convulsion, tetany

PRIMULA VULGARIS - Dropsy.

HYPERICUM - Wounds, punctures, fuzzy feelings on hands, shaking, and a paralytic weakness. Wounds of brain, spine, coccyx, fingertips, punctures from nails, thorns, wounds sensitive to touch. Painful corns and bunions.

GELSEMIUM - Sluggish mind, relaxed muscular system, limbs feel too heavy to move. Headache with functional paralysis, blurring of vision which is relieved by copious discharge of urine. Mental prostration, drooping eyelids, stage fright. Neurologic headache, nausea, vomiting, cold sweat, cold feet. Tongue coated yellowish white with fetid breath. Dry burning throat. A lot of rumbling and discomfort in the abdomen with a sudden spasmodic pain which leaves a sensation of contraction afterwards.

TABLE 7-2. Abbreviated Repertory (Continued)

CEANOTHUS - Pain in the upper left quadrant of the abdomen. Patient chilly, worse in cold weather. Depression, anorexia, "don't care" attitude.

CALENDULA - Lacerated or suppura-ting wounds. Pain, fever.

VALERIANA - Congestion of head, increased pulse, symptoms alternate between upper and limbs. Worse at noon, early afternoon, and just before midnight. Darting, tearing pains that come and go. Anxiety, hypochondriac. Goes from joyful to despair in one moment.

NAT MUR - Patient has definite character and personality. Fairly well covered and tends to be broad. Tends to be scraggly in the neck. Skin, at rest, always sallow. If excited comes in flushed and looks temporarily like a PHOSPHORUS. Flush fades and leaves patient sallow and greasy looking. Coarse greasy hair. Crack in lower lip often. Herpes on lips with cold. Walks with rapid definite movements. Often sits down shaking on putting down parcels. Worse in hot room. Much worse from consolation. Resentful if doesn't get attention, nasty if they do. "The greatest shock remedy." Hides feelings and avoids everyone. Great migraine headache remedy. Wakes with headache, gets worse until 11:00 or 12:00 noon then eases off as day gets cooler. Flashes and zig zags before eyes with headache. Headache worse with using eyes. Salt craving, likes beer, fish and occasionally milk but may have aversion to meat, coffee and fat.

NAT SULPH - Gets bronchitis in warm wet weather. Cough with dyspnea. Has to sit up quickly to get rid of sputum or lie propped up. Greenish expectoration, worse at 4-5 a.m. Left-sided pneumonia.

PHOSPHORUS - Intelligent, bright people with glint in the hair. Fine skin which flushes up quickly. Not damp skin but will sweat when nervous or with exercise. Full of apprehension if overtired. Patient thinks he is going to be ill, gets into state about business and what he has left undone. Marked fears and dreads. May fly into passion if opposed, very ashamed after. Never nurses resent-

TABLE 7-2. Abbreviated Repertory (Continued)

ment, like NAT MUR. Better with sleep. Better with rubbing. Fears dark, being alone, thunder, death and "that something will happen." Unhappy in twilight, wants reassurance. Intense thirst. Loves ice cream, loves salt, loves cold weather. Violent chest pain on coughing, better by pressure. Jaundice remedy.

PUSATILLA - Gentle, yielding type. Weeps easily, better from sympathy. Wilts in heat, can't sit in sun. Apt to have late or delayed menstruation. Often has wandering pains, rheumatism, useful in single joint rheumatism. Hates fat of any kind. Likes sweets. Very little thirst. Cough worse in evening, goes on and off until expectoration.

RHUS TOX - Greatest rheumatic and skin remedy. Lumbago worse before rain, much worse cold, very bad on getting out of bed or chair. Better after movement, much better from warmth. Very thirsty, very restless. Very good remedy for shingles when patient wants to relieve pain. Constant hot baths or applications which improves 75%. Skin complaints. Erysipelas after standing in cold wind. Patient very, very restless.

SULFUR - Untidy hair won't lie down, dirty looking, red faced, or grayish earthy appearance. Shriveled looking, "the lean dyspeptic" or the "ragged philosopher" in appearance. Redness of lips, eyelids, nostrils, anus. Ravenous hunger, often worse late morning. Sometimes emaciation.

Untidy - hates bath. Slimy diarrhea or obstinate constipation. Full of eruptions, eczema and boils. Untidy, wrong socks, burning indigestion. Desire for cold drinks and ice - worse from milk.

ARS. ALB - Headache, seven-day periodicity, Sunday headache of workers, long continued suppurations or ulcers. Old cases of gout.

Light therapy uses ultra violet light to stimulate vitamin D production, stimulate the immune system, treat sore throats, treat vaginitis, treat ringworm, athlete's foot and eczema.

Infrared light is used as an immune stimulant — this is accomplished by covering the area of interest with cloth and making a 1cm hole over an acupuncture or trigger "point." Infrared light is then directed to the hole in the cloth and allowed to redden the "point." This produces an "acute" stimulation to the "point" which causes an influx of WBCs and antibodies — any chronic process in the area will benefit from this local immune surge!!! This produces excellent results in chronic wounds, bedsores and arthritis. A standard heat lamp will produce the desired effect.

Ultra violet light is germicidal, stimulates the production of vitamin D and has "healing" effects for a variety of skin diseases and arthritis. The nice thing about the ultraviolet light used for therapy is that it is "cool" and does not produce local heat. CAUTION IS REQUIRED TO PREVENT BURNING OF YOUR EYES -- wear protective goggles or avoid looking directly at the therapy lamp tube!!!

Visible light is only five percent of the total spectrum produced by ultra violet therapy lamps. The ultra violet ray spectrum ranges between 500 and 3100 Angstrom units — 2537 Angstrom units is the "peak" intensity and is the level that produces the germicidal, erythemic and vitamin D producing effects.

Macrobiotics originated in Japan in 1946. George Ohsawa created this healing art to heal himself of tuberculosis (which he did!!); after curing himself, he opened up a macrobiotic healing center in Hiyoshi, Japan and taught from 1946 to 1952. In 1952, Ohsawa started a world lecture tour that included Africa, India, Europe and the United States. Ohsawa taught a philosophy of life and eating habits that unified people through health practices.

Macrobiotics is based on wholesome behavior and eating habits. Macrobiotic philosophy maintains that all disease and illness is caused by an imbalance of "yin" and "yang" —

"yin" - tends to be feminine, drinks, fruit, sweet, sour, hot flavors, green, blue and purple

"yang" - tends to be masculine, meat, cereals, some vegetables,hard, dense, orange or yellow

Macrobiotic diets (popularly known as the "brown rice" diet) have many reported successes with food allergies, emotional problems, chronic diseases (i.e., arthritis, diabetes, etc.) as well as long term remissions and/ or "cures" for cancer. An explanation for increased health from the macrobiotic program is that individuals who are not aware that they have gulten sensitivity (celiac disease) get benefit from eliminating wheat from their diet and begin to absorb trace minerals, vitamins and essential fatty acids.

During the height of the macrobiotic movement (1960s-1970s) in the United States, thousands of macrobiotic stores, restaurants and summer camps were opened. The most well known of Ohsawa's disciples in the United States is Michio Kushi.

Megavitamin therapy is one of the major friction points between "orthodox" medical philosophy and alternative healing arts. The "megavitamin theory" was created in 1968 and was the center of what Dr. Linus

Pauling (double Nobel Prize winner) called "orthomolecular medicine." Dr. Abram Hoffer then created "orthomolecular psychiatry."

Dr. Pauling and Dr. Hoffer used vitamins at "pharmacologic" or "therapeutic" levels for a variety of diseases with excellent results including colds, alcoholism, hyperactivity, drug addiction, osteoarthritis, neuritis, schizophrenia, depression, various psychosis and food allergies. However, as this revelation would wipe out several medical "specialties," the "orthodox" medical community refuses to publicly give a "blessing" to this form of therapy!

The doses used include five to 100 Gm of vitamin C for colds, arthritis, cancer and 3000 mg per day of niacinamide for psychosis of various types. These seem like "wild and crazy" doses when compared to the RDA of 30 mg for vitamin C and 1.5 mg for niacin!!! A variety of other nutrients are used in "mega" doses to cure or relieve acne, PMS, food allergies, arthritis, alcoholism, etc. (Table 8-1).

Naturopathy is practiced by naturopathic physicians (N.D.). What distinguishes naturopathic medicine is that its "practice" emerges from its underlying principle — FIRST DO NO HARM. Naturopathic medicine recognizes an inherent healing ability of the body. Naturopathic physicians emphasize the prevention of disease.

The "scope" of practice varies in state to state depending on the strength and oppressiveness of the "orthodox" medical lobby at the time naturopathic medicine was introduced into that state. As taught, naturopathy covers the full practice of medicine excluding major surgery (i.e., brain and chest and abdominal cavities) and the use of most legend drugs (allopathic drugs); it includes but is not limited to the following diagnostic and therapeutic modalities: nutritional science (prevention and therapy), natural hygiene, botanical medicine (herbal medicine), physical medicine (i.e., hydrotherapy, heat, cold, manipulation), oriental medicine (i.e., diagnosis, acupuncture, etc.), homeopathy, counseling, gynecology, obstetrics (natural childbirth), minor surgery, public health, immunization and all methods of laboratory and physical/clinical diagnosis. It is claimed that Hippocrates was the father of modern naturopathic medicine since he was an herbalist.

Naturopathic medicine is licensed and/or regulated by a separate board of examiners or licenses in several countries and states including England, Europe, Canada, Australia and the United States (i.e., Oregon, Washington, Washington, D.C., Arizona, Hawaii, Nevada, Florida, Connecticut, Georgia, Utah, Idaho, North Carolina, Alaska and Montana).

Negative ion therapy is the use of negatively charged air particles to prevent and cure disease. Sources of negative ions include "negative ion generators" for home and office use and frequenting forests, mountains and seashores for "free" supplies. Pure outside air has 300-1000 negatively charged ions per cubic meter of air (considerably higher levels are found at the beach) while air conditioned office or classroom air typically has 150-500. Excessive levels of positive ions in the air produces anxiety, depression and restlessness.

Negative ions 1) reduce heart rate and BP, 2) increase respiratory volume, 3) increase ciliary beat in respiratory epithelium, 4) increase efficiency of endocrine glands, 5) normalize brain rhythm, 6) reverse effects of positive ions.

Negative ion generators are particularly good for patients with inhalant allergies, asthma, respiratory disease and cystic fibrosis. Two to four treatments per day for 45 minutes each or overnight use is typical.

Osteopathy originated as a type of manipulation of body and spine to heal disease. This healing art was developed over 100 years ago by Andrew Still (an engineer) after all three of his children died at the hands of "orthodox" medicine during a meningitis outbreak. As an engineer, Still felt that disease was the result of a mechanical breakdown of the body. The American School of Osteopathy in Kirksville, Missouri was the only school for osteopaths for many years. Today it is difficult to distinguish most D.O.s from M.D.s in their "orthodox" approach — "burn, cut and poison" is the standard "allopathic" approach. There are a few exceptions among the D.O. ranks who will administer "chelation" therapy instead of rushing into bypass surgery!!!

Reflexology is an ancient Chinese and east Indian diagnostic and treatment system. The soles of the feet and palms of the hands are covered with "zones" or "points" that represent visceral organs and systems (Figure 7-2); the appearance of reflexology paralleled the appearance of acupuncture.

Ten to 30 minutes of "compression" massage is applied with the thumb or index finger. Reflexology works particularly well for physiological or functional disease. The reflexologist searches the foot or hand for "crystals" or "nodules" which are "worked out."

Rolfing is a "body therapy" (structural integration) and was named after Ida Rolf who was a graduate of biological chemistry from Barnard College, New York in 1920. In 1940, she began treating people with her technique; she worked quietly for 25 years until the 1960's "human potential" movement unveiled her treatment. In 1970, the Rolf Institute of Structural Integration was founded in Boulder, Colorado.

Rolfing is typically a deep body massage and is used to "break down" connective tissue that is pathological.

Before and after pictures are part of the process to identify posture problems and to ultimately show patients the results of treatment. Treatments tend to be very uncomfortable, but most patients feel the gains are worth the discomfort. As a result of "releasing" muscles, ligaments and connective tissue, patients get taller by 1/2 to one inch.

Urine therapy is a method of improving the patients immune system by injecting his own urine back into him. The basis of the therapy is exactly the same as the "modern" allergist uses when he injects allergens into the patient to "treat" allergies. The technique of urine injection is quite simple and can be performed at home or requested from a "user friendly" N.D., D.C., or D.O. (M.D. allergists used to use this technique for 50 years until the pharmaceutical companies discovered they make money with prepared allergens).

Urine therapy is performed by centrifuging the patient's urine and then filtering it through a "millipore" filter to eliminate the cells and bacteria that might be present. Five to ten milliliters of urine are injected subcutaneously — this injection may cause some burning which can be eliminated by adding procaine to the filtered urine.

The urine injection technique is very useful for allergies, asthma, migraine headache and arthritis. A nonspecific increase in immune capacity has been recorded in cancer patients given urine therapy.

Yoga is a Sanscrit word meaning "oneness" and is taught by a Guru ("despoiler of darkness"). Yoga is a meditational practice to "achieve mans highest potential in life." The belief is that all of mans functions can be reduced to postures or "asanas" (yoga exercises) which are designed to prevent or cure disease. Vegetarianism is a common thread to all forms of yoga:

1) Hatha yoga - health through mastery of postures

2) Montra yoga - vibrations and radiations of life

3) Karma yoga - service to others

4) Bhakti yoga - path via devotion and love

5) Layakriya yoga - sexual relationships to achieve fulfillment in life

There are numerous healing arts and alternative medical techniques not mentioned here (i.e., iridology, kinesiology or "muscle testing," magnetism, etc.) that are generally practiced and accepted by large numbers of people so feel free to learn whatever you need to for yours and your families health.

Chapter 8
Pharmacy

"From inability to let well alone; from too much zeal for the new and contempt for what is old; from putting knowledge before wisdom, science before art, and cleverness before common sense; from treating patients as cases and from making the cure of the disease more grievous than the endurance of the same, good Lord, deliver us."

— The Library of Sir Robert Hutchison *(1871 - 1960)*

The "pharmacy" or "drugstore" is an integral part of any healing art including the home "practice." Our home "practice" has two doctors so this presents advantages and disadvantages. The advantages are that it is easy to get a "second opinion" (another viewpoint on diagnosis or treatment) and we have two widely differing specialties. The disadvantages are we don't always agree on the "pharmacy" inventory so the costs can be double.

The philosophy of the "pharmacy" should be to have an "eclectic" selection of supplies and "drugs" (medicines) without having bought things that you will never use or are not potentially useful (i.e., specialized drugs or equipment for diseases no one in your family has).

I have found a large variety of file boxes (for prescriptions), log books (for inventory) and equipment (pill counting trays, mortar and pestle, blenders, etc.) at estate and garage sales that are useful in the home "pharmacy." The personal computer is an invaluable "pharmacy" tool for storing inventories, storing names and phone numbers of "suppliers" (sources of medications and drugs); be sure to include Pharmaceutical International as a source of none FDA approved medications available on a mail order basis — phone 1-800-755-4656.

One of the more interesting pieces of pharmacy furniture I have ever seen was a Chinese herb cabinet with 100 drawers for raw herbs, pills and capsules. If you are unable to find one of these wonderful cabinets immediately, a set of shelves with stack types of plastic storage bins will work for systematically storing medications. General categories of "drugs" should be available and again we prefer an "eclectic" pharmacy that would contain several approaches for the same purpose. Lock your pharmacy to secure it from children!

Pain killers:

Topical: DMSO, H_2O_2, pain gels
benzocaine: sunburn/
wound spray
herbs: demulcents, aconite,
aloe vera, camphor, eucalyptus

Oral: Tylenol caplets
tylenol-3
aspirin
Advil
herbs: aconite, arnica
chamomile, comfrey, etc.
homeopathics

Injection: procaine
xylocaine
acupuncture: needles,
pressure, "Acu-Spark"

Antibiotics:

Topical: neomycin ointment
hydrogen peroxide
"tamed" iodine soaps or
wipes
herbs: goldenseal, garlic

Oral: liquid: penicillin
tablets/capsules: tetracycline
herbs: echinacia, goldenseal garlic
hydrogen peroxide

Injection: penicillin
tetracycline

Vitamins and minerals are the backbone of any home pharmacy — they are both your "preventive medicine" and your "therapeutic" food supplements. Food supplements at RDA levels are better than nothing but will not prevent serious disease (i.e., arthritis, osteoporosis, arteriosclerosis, senile dementia, muscular dystrophy, cystic fibrosis, pyorrhea, heart attack, cancer, etc.).

"Preventive doses" of vitamin and minerals are fairly well established (Table 8-1). These are considerably higher than RDAs but not in the "megavitamin" range. There are excellent supplements available that can provide these levels without taking 25 tablets per meal.

"Megavitamin" levels of vitamins and minerals are used in extraordinary situations when your body requires large amounts of raw material to restore and replenish overworked organs and tissues (you do this for your car and air conditioning filters — why not your own body!!!). When indicated, "megavitamin" doses will be suggested for specific diseases and syndromes and ideally your mineral supplements will be from a plant-derived colloidal mineral source which are 98% absorbable (Chapter 10 — Materia Medica).

Homeopathic "remedies," Scheussler Cell Salts, Bach Flower "remedies," etc. can be kept in the "pharmacy" if you are going to spend the time and effort necessary to become proficient at their use — there is no value in purchasing medications or treatment equipment that you are not going to use.

Syrup of Ipecac can be used as an "expectorant" at the dose of 0.5 ml orally or as an "emetic" at 15-30 ml (1/2-1 tbsp.) to remove ingested poisons — follow with large volumes of water. (CAUTION: DO NOT CAUSE VOMITING FOR INGESTED CORROSIVES.)

Adrenalin should be available for shock (sudden allergic reaction to bee sting, food allergies, asthma, etc.) in the form of a bee sting kit — these are available at any commercial pharmacy.

ACE (adrenal cortical extract) sublingual drops does wonders for any kind of stress (i.e., family problems, work deadlines, chronic disease processes, final exams, etc.).

Oxygen in the form of a 30 minute supply (home tank) can save your, or another family member's or neighbor's life in case of an electric shock (stop breathing), drowning, asthma or heart attack.

Ammonia vials (smelling salts) are good for fainting or dizziness from a right cross.

Disposable supplies (i.e., bandages, lubricant jelly, gauze "sponges," cleansing wipes, "butterfly" bandages, gloves, syringes, needles, sutures, etc.) can be kept in quantities based on your family's size, lifestyle, and needs.

Cough medicines: You can use commercial nighttime cough medicines for much needed rest and use herbal "remedies" during the day or you can use steam with eucalyptus oil. You can use some very effective herbs day and night such as comfrey, garlic, licorice, ephedra, mullein.

Lastly, don't repeat the mistakes of the "orthodox" physician by "prescribing" too many medications — constant re-evaluation will prevent this!!!

Fig. 8-1. Base Line Nutritional Supplement Program for Adults*

Nutrient	RDA	True Supplement Need	30-Day Pharmacologic Daily Dose
BIOTIN	200 mcg	200 mcg	500 to 3,000 mcg
CALCIUM	800 mcg	2,000 mg	2,000 to 5,000 mg
CHLORIDE	1,700 mg	2,500 mg	500 to 2,500 mg
CHOLINE	150 mg	600 mg	500 to 1,000 mg
CHROMIUM	50 mcg	200 mcg	300 to 600 mcg
COPPER	2 mg	3 to 4 mg	4 to 6 mg
FLUORIDE	1.5 mg	1.5 mg	20 mg**
FOLIC ACID	400 mcg	1,000 mcg	15 to 20 gm
INOSITOL	75 mg	90 mg	500 to 2,000 mg
IODINE	150 mcg	250 mcg	1,000 mcg
IRON	18 mg	45 mg	50 to 100 mg
MAGNESIUM	350 mg	1,000 mg	1,000 mg
MANGANESE	2.5 mg	5 mg	2 to 50 mg
MOLYBDENUM	15 mcg	500 mcg	1,000 mcg
NIACIN	18 mg	50 mg	2,000 to 6,000 mg (time release)
PANTOTHENIC ACID	4 mg	50 mg	300 to 1,000 mg (per day)
PHOSPHORUS	800 mg	0.0	0.0
POTASSIUM	1,875 mg	5,500 mg	5,500 mg****
PYRIDOXINE	2.2 mg	50 mg	200 to 500 mg
RIBOFLAVIN	1.6 mg	50 mg	200 to 500 mg
SELENIUM	?	200 mcg	500 to 3,000 mcg
SODIUM	1,100 mg	3,300 mg	300 to 3,000 mg
SULPHUR	?	500 mg	1,000 mg
THIAMINE	1.4 mg	50 mg	200 to 500 mg
TIN	?	500 mcg	1000 mcg
VANADIUM	?	500 mcg	2 - 5 mg
VITAMIN A		5,000 IU	20,000 IU - 300,000 IU*** (beta carotene)
VITAMIN B-12	3 mcg	200 mcg	1,000 mcg
VITAMIN C	60 mg	1,000 mg	10,000 mg
VITAMIN D	400 IU	275 IU	1,000 IU
VITAMIN E	15 IU	400 IU	1,200 IU
VITAMIN K	70 mcg	140 mcg	140 mcg
ZINC	15 mg	25 mg	150 mg

* The most efficient way to get mineral supplements is in the plant derived colloidal liquid form.

** Use this level only with a prescription for osteoporosis.

*** as beta carotene

**** available in food

Chapter 9

OB/GYN

"The knife is dangerous in the hand of the wise, let alone in the hand of the fool."
— Hebrew Proverb

Contrary to the "orthodox" OB/GYN teaching and general medical thought, pregnancy is a normal biological process and not a disease! The hospitalization of women for the delivery of babies is rarely necessary (i.e., Rh, placenta previa, etc.) for safety purposes; this mania for having babies in the hospital was dreamt up by the "orthodox" OB/GYN so that they would avoid the "waste" of time at the mother-to-be's house and, therefore, see more patients in a day. This process has been taken to the extreme in modern times where the OB/GYN has his office across the parking lot from the hospital, the "patient" is monitored by nurses until the "moment of truth" (dilation of the cervix to 10 cm); the OB/GYN is then called on his beeper and he runs across the parking lot from his busy office (like OJ in the Hertz TV ads) to "catch" the baby then turn it over to pediatrician within minutes of birth and run back across the parking lot to his office to plug more "cows" (that's their term, folks!) into the parlor. So for 15 to 30 minutes of watching a normal event, he gets $1,000!!!

If the above scenario was the only transgression we could chalk it off to overconcern for their patient; however, a critical look at statistics reveals the true nature of the "orthodox" OB/GYN! If the poor lady is having her first baby (first labor is normally an 18 to 24 hour process) and without the council of her mother or grandmother, she will do anything to stop the discomfort of the contractions, anything! She is an easy mark for a salesman in a white coat and green "scrubs" who wants to get back to his office, dinner party, or get away for the ski weekend!!!. He will say, "it's in the best interest of the baby to have a caesarian section at this time as extended labor (longer than six hours in their book) can exhaust the baby." This fact is borne out by the fact that 35% of all hospital births are delivered by C-section today!!!

The 35% statistic says that either fully one third of our American women are abnormal and can't have a God-designed vaginal birth or that the OB/GYN "specialists" have found a new "fraud" that they can "hoodwink" the patient and insurance company with to max out their income for time expended (kind of like taking out your normal appendix when you go into the hospital for a checkup). As an ND in practice in Oregon, I delivered some 200 babies at home and referred one to a hospital for a C-section (that's 0.5% — maybe veterinarians know something that the human OB/GYN doesn't!!!) Lastly, to keep the cash flow up, the "orthodox" OB/GYN deems by fiat that all following babies "must be delivered by C-section because of the weakened uterine wall."

Home births are the best way to save money, bring the family together and save yours and your baby's life. More infections occur in the newborn and in women during postdelivery in the hospital than at home! It has been this way since time immemorial. Today, the United States is listed as 23rd in newborn mortality and first year survival rate compared with other industrialized nations by the WHO!!! Of the 183,955 newborns delivered at the Vienna Children's Hospital by "orthodox" doctors between 1774 and 1836, 80% died compared with 5% mortality in those delivered by midwives during the same time period!

This spectacular statistic was recorded by a young doctor (Semmelwise) who noted that the "orthodox" doctors simply didn't have the courtesy to wash their "God-like" hands between leaving the autopsy room and delivering babies. The midwives on the other hand had the basic decency to wash their hands before delivering babies. Was Semmelwise honored for this awesome discovery? No! He was committed to an insane asylum by his "colleagues" where he mysteriously died!!!

You can do your own breast self-examination, take advantage of free or reduced fee mammograms offered by hospitals (women younger than 40 should consider the increased risk of breast cancer), self-internal examination (vaginal and cervix), keep track of your cycles and periods. It is important to perform these examinations monthly so you will immediately recognize any abnormal change.

Birth control (i.e., condoms, spermicidal creams, jellies, and foams, sponges, etc.) can be obtained OTC (over the counter) from pharmacies and grocery stores (next they will show up at McDonald's) without a prescription from the "orthodox" doctor. These forms of contraception are a lot safer than IUDs (i.e., Delcon Shield) and birth control pills (i.e., deaths, blood clots, sterility). Pregnancy is easily diagnosed at home with any of the numerous HPT kits (Home Pregnancy Test) that can be purchased from the pharmacy or grocery store, as can prenatal vitamins (you should be on vitamins and minerals (i.e., baseline nutrition supplement program) if you are sexually active to prevent birth defects). Preconception supplements and prenatal supplements are cheap "insurance" against the tragedy and human misery brought about by birth defects.

You can weigh yourself, take your own blood, take your own blood pressure, test your own urine. The public health lab will run your blood test for Rh, anemia, toxoplasmosis, etc. Take a Lamaze class to understand pregnancy and labor ("orthodox" OB/GYNs don't like these classes because they can't sell you a C-section when you are informed!)

You can go to a hospital or university and ask for an ultrasound exam to determine the location of the placenta and the actual age of your baby (and rule out twins).

Except for twins, placenta previa, pelvic deformity or Rh problems, you can have your baby at home.

Weight gains from 28 to 40 pounds is normal for a pregnancy and is the additive weight of the baby, the placenta, the fluid surrounding the baby and the fetal membranes. Sudden weight gains of ten or more pounds after the 20th week of pregnancy can harold toxemia of pregnancy; the weight gain is the result of low blood protein which causes fluid retention (this is usually the result of low protein diets to keep the OB/GYN happy about weight gain). Increasing the protein intake to 120 to 200 gms per day (animal protein) will solve the problem.

You are now armed with enough data to decide if you want to have a home birth. If you choose a home birth, contact an ND (naturopathic physician), a chiropractor (state of Oregon) or a midwife for assistance.

Birth defects are our "pet peeve." If you are a sexually active woman and have been visiting an "orthodox" OB/GYN for three months, he should have prescribed a baseline nutritional supplement program for you to prevent birth defects; if not and you have had a child with a birth defect or low birth weight requiring expensive intensive care, you are within your rights to sue them for malpractice. In a review of causes of birth defects, 98% are known to be caused by nutritional deficiencies (i.e., cystic fibrosis, muscular dystrophy, heart defects, brain defects, spina bifida, cleft palates or limb defects, hernia, etc.); radiation, by contrast, causes less than 0.10% of the total birth defects since most pregnant women know to avoid x-rays during early pregnancy; teenagers have a bigger percentage of children with birth defects than do women over 40 because of generally poor eating habits, lack of supplementation programs and competition from their own critical demands for nutrients during the rapid growth and development of early puberty.

Literally billions of dollars have been spent perfecting preconception and pregnancy rations for laboratory, pet and agricultural animals that have totally eliminated birth defects. These pelleted diets provide perfect nutrition with every mouthful and totally prevent birth defects; these diets were formulated so testing on drugs would reveal any teratogenic effect (i.e., thalidomide disaster) of the drug. Again, why should a laboratory rat get treated better than our pregnant women? Again, a whole medical specialty of "orthodox" pediatrics would get wiped out so you know the answer!!!

Specific examples of serious birth defects that can be prevented include "cystic fibrosis" which is billed by the "orthodox" doctors as the "most common genetic defect" known to man for the last 40 years. In reality, "cystic fibrosis" is a selenium and fatty acid deficiency in the fetus and/or newborn breastfed infant. Maternal malabsorption of selenium from subclinical celiac disease is the initiating cause of selenium deficiency in the fetus.

Selenium deficiency in the fetus and newborn produces the classic "cystic fibrosis" lesions of the pancreas. "Cystic fibrosis" patients are born with normal lungs and have a negative "sweat test" at birth. Over the first few months of life, the infant develops a "positive sweat test" as they loose the essential fatty acids given to them by their mother as a fetus.

The "sweat test" is a test put forth in 1958 by Dr. Paul de St. Agnese of NIH as "the diagnostic test for CF" (even though he knew at that time that a "positive sweat test" was also given by eight other diseases -i.e., celiac disease, allergies, starvation, etc.).

In 1958, Dr. Klaus Schwartz reported in the Federation Proceedings (the official NIH Journal) that selenium was an essential nutrient; being a good German scientist, he recorded all tissue changes of selenium deficiency including classical changes of CF (this was a blind study as he knew nothing about CF) in the pancreas of test rats and mice.

In 1972, Cornell University showed that chicks hatched from selenium deficient hens developed classical "cystic fibrosis" of the pancreas (again they knew nothing of CF and were only studying selenium deficiency). The most amazing part of this experiment was that when selenium was given within 30 days of hatching the CF was totally cured within 21 days!!!

In 1978, I (Wallach) discovered the first agreed upon CF in nonhumans; the test animals were NASA monkeys; the diagnosis was agreed to by experts from Johns Hopkins Medical School, Emory University and the CF Foundation!!! Once they realized that this wasn't a genetic accident but CF was a recreatable selenium deficiency, they fired me with 24 hours' notice, 10 days after my wife had died. Dr. Paul de St. Agnese stated that "if anything important was to be discovered on CF, it would be in his NIH laboratory."

Since 1978, we have treated 450 CF patients with excellent results; we have essentially cured infants three months old who started on the program (they are 12 years old today) and have helped CF women have healthy pregnancies and normal babies!

Additional evidence that CF is a birth defect caused by a selenium deficiency is the results of a joint research project carried out by ourselves and research scientists from the People's Republic of China. The study was carried out with Dr. Yu, Wei Han and Dr. Yu, Feng Teng of Harbin Medical University and Dr. Gu, Bo-Qi of Shanghai First Medical University of Shanghai.

We examined the tissue of 1700 Chinese children that died of Keshan Disease (a fatal heart fibrosis of children recognized by the WHO as a selenium deficiency disease). We reasoned that if CF was truly a selenium deficiency disease, we would find at least one classic CF pancreas in a group that size (the proponents of the genetic theory postulate the CF "gene" is found in 1/2500 people — in addition CF is supposed to be a "genetic" disease of people with "middle European" backgrounds). In fact, we found that 595 or 35% had classical CF lesions of the pancreas — obviously highly significant!!! In a review of over 400 CF autopsies, 79 had Keshan Disease of the heart!!!

The most critical question has been why do some mothers get selenium deficiencies when the American diet is rich in selenium (even in selenium deficient soil areas because of widespread food importation). The answer is quite simple. Food allergies cause celiac disease type changes in the absorptive surface of the gut of the mother and the fetus which results in a malabsorption syndrome. Not only does this malabsorption syndrome cause CF but other defects as well. Breast-feeding by a selenium deficient mother further aggravates the infant's selenium deficiency.

General public distribution of the fact that maternal

malabsorption syndromes, food allergies (i.e., celiac disease) and nutritional deficiencies result in birth defects and that good nutritional supplementation and forthright aggressive treatment of food allergies will never be put forth by the "orthodox" OB/GYN or pediatricians. Remember Dr. Author F. Coco (creator of the pulse test) lamented "I am a realist, as long as the profit is in the treatment of symptoms rather than a search for causes; that's where the medical profession will go for its harvest." It's our contention that a class action suit should be brought against the perpetrators of this crime by all families with CF children born after 1958. (If this seems a bit harsh to you, consider that the AMA and individual state medical boards try to totally get rid of chiropractic of naturopathy in their state if one person is injured by an individual scoundrel).

Infertility is another common problem in Americans that is primarily a nutritional problem. Why can a farmer have 100 cows, 100 pregnancies and 100 normal calves. We have successfully tested literally hundreds of cases of infertility with nutritional revitalization of both the husband and the wife. Farmers have known the basic "truth" that the mare to be put with the stallion has to be fed special foods for 90 to 120 days prior to the actual breeding process. How can we expect conceptions in women with poor nutrition, no supplementation or malabsorption syndromes.

At a recent convention, I met a young female "orthodox" doctor who had been trying for a pregnancy for years with no success. In reviewing her lab work, we found her blood vitamin A level at 10% of normal despite supplementation — a classic case of malabsorption. You know the rest — rotation diets, find out what food allergies she has, consider celiac disease, and supplementation (120 days — BINGO! A pregnancy!)

Pregnancy Table

the date below this will be the expected day of delivery.

Jan.	1	2	3	4	5	6	7	8	9	10	11	12	13	14	15	16	17	18	19	20	21	22	23	24	25	26	27	28	29	30	31	
Oct.	**8**	**9**	**10**	**11**	**12**	**13**	**14**	**15**	**16**	**17**	**18**	**19**	**20**	**21**	**22**	**23**	**24**	**25**	**26**	**27**	**28**	**29**	**30**	**31**	**(1**	**2**	**3**	**4**	**5**	**6**	**7**	**Nov.**
Feb.	1	2	3	4	5	6	7	8	9	10	11	12	13	14	15	16	17	18	19	20	21	22	23	24	25	26	27	28				
Nov.	**8**	**9**	**10**	**11**	**12**	**13**	**14**	**15**	**16**	**17**	**18**	**19**	**20**	**21**	**22**	**23**	**24**	**25**	**26**	**27**	**28**	**29**	**30**	**(1**	**2**	**3**	**4**	**5**				**Dec.**
Mar.	1	2	3	4	5	6	7	8	9	10	11	12	13	14	15	16	17	18	19	20	21	22	23	24	25	26	27	28	29	30	31	
Dec.	**6**	**7**	**8**	**9**	**10**	**11**	**12**	**13**	**14**	**15**	**16**	**17**	**18**	**19**	**20**	**21**	**22**	**23**	**24**	**25**	**26**	**27**	**28**	**29**	**30**	**31**	**(1**	**2**	**3**	**4**	**5**	**Jan.**
Apr.	1	2	3	4	5	6	7	8	9	10	11	12	13	14	15	16	17	18	19	20	21	22	23	24	25	26	27	28	29	30		
Jan.	**6**	**7**	**8**	**9**	**10**	**11**	**12**	**13**	**14**	**15**	**16**	**17**	**18**	**19**	**20**	**21**	**22**	**23**	**24**	**25**	**26**	**27**	**28**	**29**	**30**	**31**	**(1**	**2**	**3**	**4**		**Feb.**
May	1	2	3	4	5	6	7	8	9	10	11	12	13	14	15	16	17	18	19	20	21	22	23	24	25	26	27	28	29	30	31	
Feb.	**5**	**6**	**7**	**8**	**9**	**10**	**11**	**12**	**13**	**14**	**15**	**16**	**17**	**18**	**19**	**20**	**21**	**22**	**23**	**24**	**25**	**26**	**27**	**28**	**(1**	**2**	**3**	**4**	**5**	**6**	**7**	**Mar.**
June	1	2	3	4	5	6	7	8	9	10	11	12	13	14	15	16	17	18	19	20	21	22	23	24	25	26	27	28	29	30		
Mar.	**8**	**9**	**10**	**11**	**12**	**13**	**14**	**15**	**16**	**17**	**18**	**19**	**20**	**21**	**22**	**23**	**24**	**25**	**26**	**27**	**28**	**29**	**30**	**31**	**(1**	**2**	**3**	**4**	**5**	**6**		**April**
July	1	2	3	4	5	6	7	8	9	10	11	12	13	14	15	16	17	18	19	20	21	22	23	24	25	26	27	28	29	30	31	
April	**7**	**8**	**9**	**10**	**11**	**12**	**13**	**14**	**15**	**16**	**17**	**18**	**19**	**20**	**21**	**22**	**23**	**24**	**25**	**26**	**27**	**28**	**29**	**30**	**(1**	**2**	**3**	**4**	**5**	**6**	**7**	**May**
Aug.	1	2	3	4	5	6	7	8	9	10	11	12	13	14	15	16	17	18	19	20	21	22	23	24	25	26	27	28	29	30	31	
May	**8**	**9**	**10**	**11**	**12**	**13**	**14**	**15**	**16**	**17**	**18**	**19**	**20**	**21**	**22**	**23**	**24**	**25**	**26**	**27**	**28**	**29**	**30**	**31**	**(1**	**2**	**3**	**4**	**5**	**6**	**7**	**June**
Sept.	1	2	3	4	5	6	7	8	9	10	11	12	13	14	15	16	17	18	19	20	21	22	23	24	25	26	27	28	29	30		
June	**8**	**9**	**10**	**11**	**12**	**13**	**14**	**15**	**16**	**17**	**18**	**19**	**20**	**21**	**22**	**23**	**24**	**25**	**26**	**27**	**28**	**29**	**30**	**(1**	**2**	**3**	**4**	**5**	**6**	**7**		**July**
Oct.	1	2	3	4	5	6	7	8	9	10	11	12	13	14	15	16	17	18	19	20	21	22	23	24	25	26	27	28	29	30	31	
July	**8**	**9**	**10**	**11**	**12**	**13**	**14**	**15**	**16**	**17**	**18**	**19**	**20**	**21**	**22**	**23**	**24**	**25**	**26**	**27**	**28**	**29**	**30**	**31**	**(1**	**2**	**3**	**4**	**5**	**6**	**7**	**Aug.**
Nov.	1	2	3	4	5	6	7	8	9	10	11	12	13	14	15	16	17	18	19	20	21	22	23	24	25	26	27	28	29	30		
Aug.	**8**	**9**	**10**	**11**	**12**	**13**	**14**	**15**	**16**	**17**	**18**	**19**	**20**	**21**	**22**	**23**	**24**	**25**	**26**	**27**	**28**	**29**	**30**	**31**	**(1**	**2**	**3**	**4**	**5**	**6**		**Sept.**
Dec.	1	2	3	4	5	6	7	8	9	10	11	12	13	14	15	16	17	18	19	20	21	22	23	24	25	26	27	28	29	30	31	
Sept.	**7**	**8**	**9**	**10**	**11**	**12**	**13**	**14**	**15**	**16**	**17**	**18**	**19**	**20**	**21**	**22**	**23**	**24**	**25**	**26**	**27**	**28**	**29**	**30**	**(1**	**2**	**3**	**4**	**5**	**6**	**7**	**Oct.**

Chapter 10

Materia Medica

> *"I firmly believe that if the entire materia medica as now used would be sunk to the bottom of the sea, it would be all the better for mankind — and all the worse for the fishes."*
>
> — Oliver Wendell Homes

The best part about "playing doctor" is the actual "treatment" of yourself or others. As with everything, "when all else fails — read the directions." It is recommended that you read and learn the preceding chapters before embarking on this section (otherwise you might wind up like the "orthodox" doctor).

It was said by Ben Franklin that "an ounce of prevention is worth a pound of cure" so this chapter is designed to give preventative programs as well as therapies. We often hear our patients say "I just can't take all of these supplements and medications!!! " to which we reply "taking supplements is a small exchange, cheap insurance if you will, in return for the prevention of a major disease such as heart disease, arthritis, or cancer." We go to a great deal of expense and effort to prevent major automobile wear by changing oil, filters and transmission fluid — why not treat our bodies as well as we do our "beamer" (BMW). Preventive maintenance of our bodies can cost as little as $1 to $5 per day depending on whether you want a $10,000 or $50,000 "insurance' policy (smoking and drinking cost considerably more!!!).

A baseline of vitamins and minerals are essential to preventive health programs; it is impossible to obtain enough nutrition from our food to reach the maximum genetic potential of 130 health-filled years. Therefore, we recommend taking supplements at preventive levels (Fig. 8-1) in divided doses t.i.d. (three times per day) to keep blood levels elevated for at least 12 hours per day. All recommended supplemental levels of nutrients for specific diseases are to be taken in addition to the base prevention amounts.

References for this book, including those for this chapter, will be found at the end for two reasons: 1) to prevent the book from being so large you couldn't carry it and 2) keep the cost down — one reason medical books cost $120 is that there are more pages of references than there are pages of facts and "how to" information. The information in this book represents five college degrees — a total of 24 years of college — and 50 years of combined research and clinical experience. In addition, no less than 200 books have been "predigested" for you in hopes of saving you time and expense. Those who wish to spend the time and effort to follow up one or more points in more detail will be able to do so with some ease as we have chosen a few books that are comprehensive reviews (from there you can go to thousands of journal articles if you so desire).

A last bit of advice is to avoid problems in diagnosis and treatment by spending some time confirming your "diagnosis" and reviewing the "treatments" — don't become like the "orthodox" doctors and "shoot from the hip" in a trial and error type of "practice." Now armed with all this information, we are in a position to take back control of our own health. Let the revolution begin!!!

LET'S PLAY DOCTOR!!!

ABRASIONS (scrapes): clean wounds with soap and water to remove gross dirt and debris. Disinfect wounds with H_2O_2 (hydrogen peroxide). Wounds may be bathed in a variety of herbal washes or poultice — our choice is aloe, plantain (Plantago major) or comfrey (Symphytum officinale) colloidal silver is useful here. Vitamin C orally to bowel tolerance (anywhere from 1-5 grams). Covering abrasions with nonstick dressings will help prevent infection.

ABSCESS (boil): bring abscess to "a head" (a soft point in the center) with a compress or poultice (sitz bath if near the anus or buttock) using a 3% solution of boric acid; herbal alternatives include echinacea (Echinacea angustifolia) or sand sagebrush (Artemisia fififolia). Once the abscess opens (by itself or with a sterile needle or blade) it can be flushed clean using a syringe filled with any of the above solutions. If large enough, the resulting cavity can be filled with gauze (umbilical "tape" is particularly good for this purpose) soaked with any of the above solutions. If the abscess cavity contains bits of puss or dead tissue, it can be flushed with H_2O_2. The cavity will gradually fill with "granulation tissue" leaving no trace of the cavity. Vitamin C orally to bowel tolerance.

ABSENCE ATTACKS (petit mal): patient stops what he is doing and rapidly blinks eyes then starts the activity again where he left off. Treatment should include choline 4 gm/day; taurine 500 mg t.i.d.; dimethyl glycine 100 mg b.i.d., phosphytidyl choline and B-6 100-300 mg/day.

ACHALASIA (megaesophagus): enervation of the

esophagus resulting in failure of cardiac (lower sphincter) sphincter to open. A tendency to regurgitate undigested food is a common sign. Small liquid meals and air swallowing can sometimes relieve this condition. Night time elevation of head of the bed will reduce risk of vomiting while asleep. Surgery may be required to relieve severe cases.

ACHLORHYDRIA (loss of stomach acid): contrary to belief stress will result in loss of stomach acid production. Achlorhydria is also a natural process of aging (perhaps the most significant aging phenomenon) so much so that 75% of people over the age of 50 years require supplementation. Symptoms include "burp/belch and bloat" because the absence of acid in the stomach allows intestinal bacteria and yeast (Candida albicans) to enter the stomach and ferment high carbohydrate foods (i.e. juice, fruit, breads, etc.). Failure to deal with achlorhydria will result in B-12, calcium and protein deficiencies and the onset of new food allergies as a result of absorption of partially digested polypeptides (relatively large protein fragments).

Treatment includes supplementation of betaine HCl at the rate of 75-250 mg 15-20 minutes before each meal. In the absence of betaine HCl 1-2 oz. of vinegar with English bitters (Gentian) may be taken before meals. Additionally, plant derived colloidal minerals tonify the stomach and increase its ability to produce stomach acid.

ACNE (acne rosacea/acne vulgaris): a frequent skin disease in teenagers and sometimes associated with PMS. Acne is characterized by papules, pustules, superficial puss-filled cysts and deep puss-filled canals. Acne is primarily the result of an essential fatty acid deficiency with a concurrent intake of too much saturated fat. Eliminate fast foods and other sources of fat and sugar. Check out the probability of food allergies (i.e., wheat, milk, soy); betaine HCl and pancreatic enzymes are of considerable benefit; essential fatty acids are a must (flaxseed oil - 1 tbsp. b.i.d.); vitamin A 300,000 units/day (as beta carotene) for five months; B-6 100 mg t.i.d.; zinc 50 mg t.i.d.; vitamin E oil may be applied topically to acne lesions; ultra violet light directly to areas of acne for 1-6 minutes.

ADRENAL GLAND EXHAUSTION (stress): characterized by fatigue and inability to cope with diseases or every day stresses. Adrenal exhaustion directly affects your ability to resist disease or heal a current disease. An adrenal function test can be performed in the following manner. Take base blood pressure in a lying down position after five minutes then stand up suddenly-pulse should increase by a minimum of ten points; if not, your adrenals need help. Concurrent signs and symptoms may include colitis, ulcers and low WBC count.
Treatment of adrenal exhaustion includes ACE (adrenal cortical extract) ten drops of a standard solution sublingually or 3-5 ml IV; vitamin C to bowel tolerance; and zinc 25-50 mg t.i.d. Don't forget to remove the stress.

AGE SPOTS (Liver spots): These unsightly brown spots are caused by rancid fat from cell walls accumulating under the skin — if you have ten on the back of your hand, you have thousands in your brain, heart, liver, kidney, lungs, etc. They interfere with cell function, shorten your life and are a red flag warning for high risk of cancer and heart disease (i.e. cardiomyopathy). The nice things about age spots is that they are reversible and when they go away on the outside, they are going away on the inside.

Treatment includes eliminating all fried foods, vegetable oils (i.e., salad dressing, cooking oils, margarine, etc.) and sugar from the diet; also take selenium at 500 mcg, vitamin E at 1, 200 IU and all 90 essential nutrients.

AGREEABLE ATTITUDE: usually a disagreeable attitude is the result of food allergies or hypoglycemia (sometimes from poor training while growing up!); if so these must be dealt with specifically.
Treatment should include plantain (Plantago lanceolata) orally t.i.d., avoidance of sugar in all forms (i.e., alcohol, deserts, sugar, juices, fruits, etc.), avoidance of caffeine; essential fatty acids 1 tbsp. b.i.d., chromium and vanadium at 50-100 mcg each t.i.d.

AIDS (autoimmune deficiency syndrome): thought to be caused by the HIV virus. This disease may lay dormant for three to ten years before causing overt symptoms and death. Signs are very low WBC counts especially T-cells; coughing and susceptibility to a variety of diseases including Pneumo-cystis carnii pneumonia, Karposi's Sarcoma and a variety of secondary bacterial and viral infections. This disease is transmitted by oral, vaginal and anal sex, common needles used for IV drugs, contaminated hospital and dental equipment, commercially prepared blood products, and immunotoxic lubricants.
At this point (1992) prevention is the "magic bullet" for AIDS. Avoid IV "recreational drugs," use unlubricated condoms for sex with partners with unknown sexual histories. Avoid anal sex. Once AIDS is contracted, a vigorous program of antiviral medications (i.e., Ribavirin and Isoprinosin) and immune support (Levamisol , hydrazine sulfate) are indicated. Vitamin C to bowel tolerance, 300,000 IU of vitamin A per day as beta carotene, 50 mg

zinc t.i.d., ACE (adrenal cortical extract) 10 drops t.i.d. sublingual, selenium 1000 mcg/day orally or by injection, vitamin E 1000 IU/day, herbs such as garlic (Allium sativum), evening primrose oil (Oenothera biennis) and goldenseal (Hydrastis canadensis) may be of value. Long-term remission can be expected but "cure" is not available. An unknown in this protocol is Levamisol which may be the immune modulator that everyone is looking for. Injectable thymus monthly at 3-5 cc after four initial daily injections of 3-5 cc.

ALCOHOLISM: considered to be an addictive allergy complicated by hypoglycemia and vitamin/mineral malnutrition. Rotation elimination diets and hypoglycemia diets are essential. Don't forget the baseline vitamin/mineral supplements. Calcium (2000 mg) and magnesium (1000 mg) per day; essential fatty acids 5 mg t.i.d. and B-6 100 mg b.i.d.; chromium 250 mcg/day is essential to solve the hypoglycemia problem; bioflavonoids (catechin) 1 gram/day and amino acids (i.e., DL-phenylananine).
Take 1 oz. plant derived colloidal minerals every time craving for alcohol occurs.

ALLERGIES: can be caused by food, inhalant allergens (i.e., pollens, smoke, molds, etc.) or chemicals (i.e., perfume, formalin, etc.). Diagnosis can be made using the pulse test, diet diary/ challenge and cytotoxic test. Symptoms vary widely from urticaria (skin rash with itching) from strawberries or fish; headaches from perfume; tachycardia (fast heart rate) or palpitations (most allergies-MSG); or paranoia from sugar, etc; asthma-like syndrome from sulfite (food preservative on raisins, apricots, etc.).
Avoidance is the most effective "cure," however, this may

be impractical. Autoimmune urine therapy using five to ten ml of filtered urine subcutaneously every other day for five to eight treatments) using a 0.22 micron millipore filter. Vitamin C to bowel tolerance; bioflavonoids (rutin, catechin, quercetin); 300,000 IU of vitamin A as beta carotene per day; zinc 50 mg t.i.d., essential fatty acids 1 tbsp. b.i.d., rotation diets.

ALLERGIC SHINERS: are the purplish/ black discolorations under the lower eyelids of individuals with allergies. They will appear within minutes of ingestion or inhalation of an allergen. Allergic shiners may take as much as 12 hours to three days to disappear after avoidance of allergenic substance. Allergic shiners are a good diagnostic tool (i.e., allergic shiners in a hyperactive child, heart disease, cancer, etc.). Avoidance of the allergen or allergens is the only "cure" for allergic shiners.

ALZHEIMERS DISEASE: is a physician caused disease in which those afflicted suffer from a progressive loss of memory with difficulties with arousal and motor function appearing in the later stages of the disease. Identified in 1979 it appears to be due to a cholesterol deficiency. Treatment should include germanium IM 5 ml of standard solution every other day for 24 days followed by oral germanium at 150/mg b.i.d.; hydergine 6-12 mg/ day; piracetam/choline 1.6 grams q.i.d.; vasopressin (Diapid) at a rate of one whiff in each nostril q.i.d. which delivers a total daily dose of 12-16 units of U.S.P. Posterior Pituitary; centrophenoxine (Lucidril) 6.2-8.0 gram/ day. Lecithin at 2,500 mg t.i.d. is very useful at all stages (phosphatydil choline is more efficient). Don't forget the baseline nutritional supplements (including colloidal minerals), betaine HCl and pancreatic enzymes 75-200 mg t.i.d., oral and IV H_2O_2; 200 mg vitamin B-1 t.i.d., vitamin E at 1200 iu daily and IV chelation will be of value. Eat soft-scrambled eggs every day and 72 oz. red meat each month to replace cholesterol.

ALOPECIA (baldness): loss of hair which can occur locally or present as total hair loss. Male pattern baldness, female pattern baldness and alopecia universalis are examples.
Monoxidil and Retin-A creams will aid some male and female pattern baldness if treated early in the process and use is maintained. Deficiencies of colloidal tin have been shown to cause male pattern baldness in lab animals (one of us — Wallach — has had considerable hair regrowth following the use of plant derived liquid colloidal tin). Alopecia that occurs with eczema is often caused by essential fatty acid deficiency and will respond to IV interlipids and/ or oral flaxseed oil at the rate of 1 tbsp. b.i.d.; zinc at 50 mg t.i.d. Elimination of wheat and cow's milk from the diet will increase the rate of recovery. Betaine HCl and pancreatic enzymes at 75-200 mg t.i.d. 15-20 minutes before meals are a must.

AMBLYOPIA: a type of blindness that can be caused by B-12 deficiency or tobacco smoking. B-12 IM at a rate of 1000 mcg/day for a total of 20,000 mcg usually effects a "cure." Avoid tobacco smoke.

AMOEBIASIS: is an amoebic dysentery caused by Entamoeba hystolytica. Diagnosis is dependent upon finding the parasite in a stool examination. Examination of 3-6 samples may be necessary to find the organisms especially if diarrhea has been chronic. The use of the low power lens on the microscope will often allow you to observe the "amoebic" movement; bloody mucus has the highest concentration of the parasite.

Treatment should be symptomatic to relieve diarrhea and reduce the loss of protein and electrolytes. Metronidazole at the rate of 750 mg orally t.i.d. for 10 days for adults and 12-17 mg/day t.i.d. orally for children is the treatment of choice.

AMENORRHEA: is the lack of, or stopping of, the menstrual period. Many factors are involved in a normal "period" including the requirement of a 20% body fat level (trim athletes and very slim ladies stop cycling). Amenorrhea commonly occurs in very slim women athletes, dieters and anorexics, a weight gain of 10-15 pounds will "jump-start" the cycle and a "period" will result. In many cases, increased levels of zinc at a rate of 50 mg t.i.d. will result in onset of the "period." Essential fatty acids are very useful in the form of flaxseed oil at the rate of 1 tbsp. t.i.d. Herbal stimulus can be effected with saffron (Crocus sativus) as a tea, black cohosh or squawroot (Cimicifuga racemosa) as a fluid extract and marigold (Calendula officinalis).

ANAPHYLAXIS: is an explosive allergic reaction ranging from urticaria to respiratory distress and vascular collapse. This "shock" type of reaction can occur as the result of allergies to foods (i.e., shellfish), insect stings (i.e., bee stings) or drugs (i.e., penicillin) and usually occurs in 1-15 minutes after exposure. Avoidance of exposure is the best preventative.
Immediate injection with adrenaline (epinephrine) from a "bee sting" kit is the treatment of choice and, in many cases, will be lifesaving.

ANAL ABSCESS: and anal fissures are caused by constipation and frequent passage of large hard stools; they may occur at the same time with hemorrhoids. Painful red swellings at or near the anal opening are characteristic. These may be opened with a blade or by soaking in hot sitz baths of 3% boric acid. A poultice of echinacea (Echinacea angustifolia) may be applied directly to the abscess to disinfect and help to bring it to a "point" so it can be opened. Flushing the opened abscess with 3% H_2O_2 will clean out the puss and disinfect the wound.

ANEMIA: is a lack of blood from many possible causes including hemorrhage, infections and/or nutritional deficiencies. Betaine HCl orally at 75-200 mg t.i.d. 15-20 minutes before meals is required to assure absorption of B-12; liver extract orally or IM; nutritional support with iron 20 mg; B-12 1000 mcg per day for 20 days; folic acid 15 mg for 20 days; copper 2 mg; zinc 50 mg t.i.d.; B-2 50 mg b.i.d.; B-5 50 mg t.i.d.; B-6 50 mg b.i.d. for 20 days; vitamin C to bowel tolerance; Vitamin E 800-1200 IU per day; selenium 500 mcg/day; and essential fatty acids at a rate of 5 gram t.i.d. Herbs including sweet cicely (Myrrhis odorata) and marsh marigold (Coltha palustris).

ANEURYSM: is a "bubble" or "balloon" in the wall of an artery (much like a "balloon" in a weak tire) which can cause pressure on an organ like a tumor or burst causing sudden death by hemorrhage (i.e., subdural hemorrhage or stroke). Aneurysms are most frequently caused by copper deficiency which results in weakened elastic fibers; copper supplementation may not "cure" or repair an aneurysm but can prevent them at the rate of 2-4 mg/day (be sure you are absorbing). Surgery will be required for existing aneurysms (we do have one aortic aneurysm that has been corrected with copper supplementation and confirmed by x-ray).

ANGINA: is a sharp debilitating pain in the center front

of the chest from arterial disease in the heart which reduces the heart's oxygen supply. Symptoms may appear after strenuous exercise or after a meal. The allopathic approach is the "coronary bypass" surgery which after 20 years study has failed to prevent second heart attacks or to extend life (it does extend the financial portfolio of the cardiovascular surgeon!)
Chelation, either IV with H_2O_2 and calcium EDTA or orally with vitamin/mineral supplements can effect a cure over a period of time. Avoid sugar, caffeine and cigarette smoke. Exercise in the form of walking for 30 minutes each day is very helpful. Calcium (2000 mg/day) and magnesium (800 mg/day), essential fatty acids can help prevent progress of current disease and reduce vitamin D intake from the sun and supplements. Nitroglycerine sublingual capsules and time-release transdermal patches are very useful in relieving symptoms. English hawthorn (Crataegus oxyacantha) is specific for angina by increasing the blood flow through coronary arteries. Lifestyle changes and supplementation can reverse cardiovascular disease!

ANOREXIA (appetite loss): can be caused by stress, malnutrition, shock and injury, ANOREXIA NERVOSA is thought by "orthodox" medicine to be a psychiatric disease, however, it now appears that it is a manifestation of a severe food allergy (i.e., "I always feel better when I don't eat and feel bad when I eat"). Deficiencies of zinc and lithium are associated with anorexia. Elimination diets and pulse tests are useful in finding the offending food (i.e., cow's milk, wheat, eggs, corn).
Treatment should include betaine HCl and pancreatic enzymes at a rate of 150-250 mg/day t.i.d. (don't forget the baseline vitamin/mineral supplement). Herbs are excellent appetite stimulants: buckbean or marsh trefoil

(Menyanthes trifoliata); centaury (Centaurium umbellatum); sweet flag or calamus (Acorus calamus); yellow gentian (Gentiana lutea) — all of the herbal preparations should be taken before meals. In the case of ANOREXIA NERVOSA, autoimmune urine therapy is indicated.

ANOSMIA (loss of smell): can temporarily be caused by colds or rhinitis (nasal inflammation from colds or allergy). Chronic loss of the sense of smell is the result of a zinc deficiency. In the case of injury, stroke or tumor, zinc will not be effective.
Zinc supplement at the rate of 50 mg t.i.d. is very effective in returning the sense of smell.

ANXIETY (panic attacks): affects women twice as frequently as men. When one examines the total hormone biorhythm charts of women, this fact cannot be a surprise. The base cause can be either a food allergy reaction (i.e., corn, cow's milk, etc.) or a severe reactive hypoglycemic reaction often referred to as a "crash and burn" curve because the down slope on the glucose curve is almost vertical. Concurrent PMS can make this a very perplexing situation. Do a pulse test to eliminate allergies and a six-hour GTT.
Treatment should include avoidance of caffeine and sugar in all forms (fruit, juices, etc.): chromium 200-300 mcg/day; B-6 100 mg t.i.d.; B-3 450 mg t.i.d. as time-release tablets; B-1, B-2, and B-5 at the rate of 50 mg t.i.d.; L-tryptophan 10 grams t.i.d.; calcium 2000 mg/day and magnesium at 800 mg/day. Betaine HCl 100-250 t.i.d. before meals; herbs including valerian (Valerian officinalis) can be of value.

APHTHOUS STOMATITIS (canker sores): is often a

symptom of food sensitivities or allergies. An elimination/ rotation diet or a pulse test can identify the offending foods – gluten free diets are frequently effective. Folic acid at 5 mg t.i.d.; B-12 at 1000 mcg/day; iron at 15 mg/day; zinc at 50 mg t.i.d. are effective adjuncts to avoidance diets.

ARSENIC TOXICITY: is a frequent result of pollution from herbicides, slug poisons, etc. Hair analysis is the best way to determine if toxic levels of arsenic are present. Symptoms are widely varied and include: alopecia, constipation, confusion, delayed healing dermatitis, diarrhea, drowsiness, edema, fatigue, GI complaints, headache, burning and tingling, muscle pain, neuropathy, numbness, pruritis, seizures, stomatitis, weakness. Avoid oils during treatment as they promote absorption of arsenic; identify source of arsenic and eliminate it; IV chelation is very effective in removing the body load of arsenic as is the oral use of colloidal selenium.

ARTERIOSCLEROSIS (hardening of the arteries) is the result of fibrosis of the smooth muscle in the walls of elastic arteries (i.e., aorta, coronary, pulmonary, carotid, cerebral, brachial and femoral). The elevated "lesions" produce eddies which produce lipid and calcium depositions. Elevated blood cholesterol is considered to be a significant risk factor. It is of interest that vitamin D is made from cholesterol in our bodies! This becomes significant when we realize that the toxic affect of vitamin D is angiotoxicity (the target tissue of vitamin D toxicity is the elastic arteries vessels) and the specific result is fibrosis of the vascular smooth muscle and calcification of the blood vessel wall -- fatty deposits soon follow!!! It is a crime that the "orthodox" doctors do not give this as much press coverage as heart transplants. Again this information would wipe out a medical specialty, so they keep it a secret!!!

Symptoms of arteriosclerosis include angina, headaches, loss of memory, breathlessness, leg cramps ("claudication") in the early stages and death from stroke and thrombotic type "heart attack" in the final stages.

Treatment includes IV chelation with EDTA and H_2O_2, oral chelation, oral supplementation with vitamin/mineral supplements that include plant derived colloidal minerals. In addition to the baseline nutritional supplements, vitamin C to bowel tolerance; exercise (to increase the caliber of your arteries); high fiber diets that tend towards vegetarian diets low in animal fat; essential fatty acids including salmon oil and flaxseed oil 5 gm t.i.d.; useful herbs include artichoke (Cynara scolymus), bears garlic (Allium ursinum), European mistletoe (Viscum album); and garlic (Allium sativum).

ARTHRITIS (rheumatism): is a devastating degenerative disease of the joints. Symptoms of joint pain, swelling and deformative changes are typical. The cause of arthritis is listed as unknown by "orthodox" medicine and treatment is of the "take two aspirins and learn to live with it" — prednisone (a synthetic cortisone) is used to treat symptoms. In fact, arthritis is a complex of nutritional deficiencies — in the case of rheumatoid arthritis, a chronic infection with a *Mycoplasma spp.* is the overt cause. Again, if the truth were released the "orthodox" doctors would loose an entire specialty in short order, so they keep it a secret.

A dietary calcium/phosphorus ratio of 2:1 is ideal yet is impossible to attain in an unsupplemented diet. A vegetarian diet gets close but is complicated by "phytates" (a natural chelating substance found in plants) which makes even supplemented calcium unavailable. The calcium/phosphorus ratios of food items is consistent:

FOOD	CALCIUM	PHOSPHORUS
grain	1	8
red meat	1	12
organ meat *(liver, kidney)*	1	44
fish	1	12
carbonated drinks	1	8

It is easily seen that none of the calcium/phosphorus ratios of the basic foods are anywhere near correct. These increase the calcium loss from the body including the bones and teeth. The more meat you eat, the more calcium supplementation you need; it is quite simple — veterinarians know this but we suppose that "orthodox" physicians believe that if a "truth" will wipe out a medical specialty, it must be ignored or kept a secret!!!

Treatment of arthritis should include calcium at 2000 mg/day and more if you eat meat two or three times per day; magnesium at 800-1000 mg/day; cartilage or chondroitin sulfate (gelatin) at 1000 mg t.i.d.; for rheumatoid arthritis, add tetracycline at 250 mg q.i.d., or H_2O_2 to deal with the Mycoplasma. IV chelation with EDTA and H_2O_2 is very helpful! Vitamin C to bowel tolerance, B-6 100 mg b.i.d.; B-3 450 mg b.i.d. as time-release capsules. Vitamin E at 1000 IU/day. Copper at 2 mg/day (may be absorbed from a copper bracelet); selenium 300 mcg/day; zinc 50 mg t.i.d.; plant derived colloidal minerals are 98% absorbable and give excellent results!

Rotation elimination diets can help when food allergies aggravate or precipitate symptoms. Autoimmune urine therapy is very useful for all types of arthritis especially those aggravated by food allergies. DMSO or pain gels are useful in reducing inflammation and pain when applied topically. Herbs including licorice (Glycyrrhiza glabra), poison ivy (Rhus toxicodendron) and alfalfa (powder or sprouts) are useful adjuncts to arthritis treatment programs.

ASTHMA: is a respiratory disease that is characterized by sudden onset with closure of bronchial tubes by spasmodic muscles. ATOPIC ASTHMA has eczema as a feature along with the respiratory disease. This is a disease of malabsorption with essential fatty acid deficiencies and deficiencies of manganese and magnesium.
Treatment should include betaine HCl, pancreatic enzymes and ox bile at 75-200 mg each t.i.d. before meals. Autoimmune urine therapy; essential fatty acids at 5 gm t.i.d. and colloidal mineral suspensions that contain magnesium and manganese. Herbs are very useful for treating asthma with some caution when you have allergies to plants — useful plants include: honeysuckle (Lonicera caprifolium), jaborandi (Pilocarpus jaborandi), leaks (Allium porrum), garlic (Allium sativum), evening primrose oil or fluid extract (Oenothera biennia). A variety of standard "inhalers" are available to cope with sudden attacks.

ATHEROSCLEROSIS: see ARTERIOSCLEROSIS

ATOPIC DERMATITIS (eczema): is part of the "atopic" patient syndrome which includes asthma, alopecia (hair loss) and lowered immune response. This syndrome is one of malabsorption of essential fatty acids and can include emotional symptoms similar to PMS and hypoglycemia or diabetes as a result of malabsorption of chromium. The malabsorption is usually the result of a "celiac" disease type change in the small intestinal lin-

ing rather than dietary deficiency. Do a pulse test to determine food allergies.
Treatment should include a rotation elimination diet (usually a pulse test will reveal cow's milk, wheat or soy products to be the culprits); autoimmune therapy is very useful; supplementation should include essential fatty acids as flaxseed oil at 1 tbsp. b.i.d., vitamin E at 1000 IU/day. If malabsorption is a major problem, the fatty acids may be taken as interlipids IV.

ATHLETES FOOT: is actually a form of "ringworm" caused by the fungus Tinea pedis. Treatment includes hydrotherapy in baths of 3% boric acid alternating with vinegar baths. Supplements include zinc at 50 mg t.i.d., 300,000 units of vitamin A/day as beta carotene and B-6 at 100 mg b.i.d.
Various commercial athletes foot products are available as creams, sprays and powders — we prefer Desenex.

ATTENTION DEFICIT DISORDER (ADD/ADHD, Hyperkinetic): characterized as hyperactivity and inability to concentrate, cognate and retail information. Many affected are disruptive, mean and cruel to other children and small animals.
ADD and ADHD individuals (children and adults) are sensitive to sugar (natural and processed) they way some people are sensitive to alcohol. This sugar effect ranges from narcolepsy (hyperinsulinemia coma), ADD/ADHD to downright madness and criminal behavior.
The standard medical approach to ADD/ADHD is to prescribe Ritalin® or Prozac to chemically subdue the ADD/ADHD victim. The side effects of these drugs are significant and include biochemical and emotional addiction, drooling, drowsiness and explosive emotions (violence, suicide, etc.)

Treatment must include complete removal of alcohol and sugar (natural and processed) from the diet and educating the ADD/ADHD victim that there is a connection between sugar consumption and negative behavior. The whole family must eat the same way if this is to be successful! Plant derived colloidal lithium, chromium and vanadium are specific supplements to be taken — best to take all 90 essential nutrients.

AUTOIMMUNE DISORDERS: of all kinds from kidney disease to rheumatoid arthritis (the autoimmune aspect appears as a secondary event rather than the cause as the "orthodox" doctor would have you believe) can be benefited by nutritional support. Essential fatty acids are of great value and may be taken alternately as salmon oil and flaxseed oil at the rate of 5 grams t.i.d.; vitamin E at 1000 IU/day; 300,000 IU of vitamin A as beta carotene; vitamin C to bowel tolerance; zinc at 50 mg t.i.d.; and selenium at 300-1000 mcg/day. Injectable thymus at 2-5 cc/day is very useful. (See AIDS)

AUTISM: is characterized by resistance to change, repetitive acts and learning/speech disorders. Concurrent food allergies and hypoglycemia markedly aggravate the presentation of autism. Each must be dealt with as a separate entity if real progress is to be made. (Don't forget the baseline vitamin/minerals.)
Treatment should include avoidance of sugar and food allergens; supplementation should include calcium and magnesium at double the supplement rate; B-6 at five times the RDA for weight and age; and chromium for the hypoglycemia; autoimmune urine therapy can be very useful.

BACKACHE: is usually a muscle strain from overwork

and/or a "subluxation" (a malalignment of vertebrae) resulting from a fall, auto accident or improper lifting technique. On occasion, a serious case of constipation will cause a "backache" from impacted stool or pressure from gas. Eighty-five percent of adult Americans get back problems, plant derived colloidal minerals have been reported to prevent and reverse back problems without surgery.

Prevention includes proper lifting technique (straight back and bend knees), strengthening exercises, proper nutrition including calcium (2000 mg) and magnesium (800 mg), high fiber diets and eight glasses of water per day.

Treatment includes massage, chiropractic, hydrotherapy and poultices of herbs including comfrey (Symphytum officinale) and arnica (Arnica montana).

BAD BREATH: can be dealt with by basic care. Use a good anti-tartar toothpaste, hydrogen peroxide tooth gel, floss upon awakening and after meals, use a hydrogen peroxide mouthwash; parsley may be used after each meal; zinc at 50 mg t.i.d.

BALDNESS (thinning hair): see ALOPECIA. Colloidal tin is reported to be effective!

BEDSORES: result from pressure of body weight in areas of poor circulation — usually in areas of bony prominences. Massage, sponge baths and ultra violet light are good preventive therapies. Topical applications can include zinc oxide ointment, aloe vera ointment, vitamin E oil and DMSO; eucalyptus (Eucalyptus globulus), wild carrot, (Daucus carota) and comfrey (Symphytum officinale) may all be used topically and/or in poultices to encourage granulation tissue formation and healing.

BEDWETTING: is a complex syndrome of children and teenagers. It can be the result of food sensitivities or hypoglycemia. Compare what happens when the "patient" eats complex carbohydrates or ice cream and cookies before bed. Pulse tests and diet diaries with elimination diagnostic diets will be revealing.
Kids who bedwet, play with fire and are cruel to other kids an animals are potential mass murderers and serial killers — this is a serious problem not to be treated lightly. Treatment includes chromium and vanadium at 50-150 mcg/day, cranberry juice 4 oz. b.i.d. and calcium/magnesium (2000 mg/800 mg). Avoidance of sugar, simple sugars (i.e., honey, sweet juices, fruit, etc.) and allergenic foods (i.e., milk and sugar being the most common).

BEE STINGS: is a painful "sting" caused by the "injection" of bee venom (formaldehyde). Pain gels, DMSO or Caladryl lotions are very effective in relieving the pain. On occasion an individual becomes sensitive or "allergic" to the bee venom -- when this happens a potentially life threatening "shock" situation exists. Prevention is limited to avoidance of bee stings.

Treatment for individuals deemed sensitive to bee stings is limited to the use of adrenaline (epinephrine) from a "bee sting" kit.

BENIGN PROSTATIC HYPERPLASIA: is perhaps the most common infirmity of aging in the human male. More than 500,000 American males are afflicted each year. As the prostate enlarges with age, the tight outer capsule prevents the gland from expanding outwardly so it squeezes down on the neck of the bladder thus producing the well recognized symptoms of "frequency" and "urgency." The prostate is an internal gland that can be "palpated" (felt) with the gloved finger. If you are going to do this, it is important to examine the prostate monthly like a woman examines her breast monthly. The normal prostate is firm like an orange and about the size of a walnut – it is found at a depth in the rectum that is just comfortably in reach for the index finger.

Benign prostatic hypertrophy produces a uniform enlargement that may be hard in "acute" enlargement or "boggy" in chronic enlargement. Tumors, either benign or malignant tend to be irregular and nodular. PSA may be elevated.

Benign prostatic hypertrophy is treated with zinc at 50 mg t.i.d., essential fatty acids as flaxseed oil at 1 tbsp. t.i.d., high fiber diets including pumpkin seeds and alfalfa, 300,000 IU vitamin A as beta carotene per day, vitamin C to bowel tolerance, chlorophyll (best source is alfalfa), amino acids (glycine, alanine and glutamic acid) at five grams each daily for 90 days, hydrogen peroxide (20 drops per oz. of aloe juice) at 1 oz. b.i.d., cranberry juice at two pints per day, herbs including saw palmetto (Sarenoa serrulata) and selenium at 250 mcg t.i.d.

BELLS PALSY: is the sudden drooping of one side of the face due to an inflammation, swelling or squeezing of the "facial" nerve (the 7th cranial nerve as it passes through the skull). Bells palsy is often mistaken for a stroke because of the sudden onset. Numbness and partial or total loss of muscular control on the affected side are typical signs and symptoms. Treated properly, there can be as much as an 80% chance of significant recovery. Treatment is B-12 at 1000 mcg/day for a total of 20,000 mcg; calcium/ magnesium at 2,000 mg and 800 mg per day; essential fatty acids at 5 gm t.i.d. and American ginseng (Panax quinquefolius). Colloidal minerals are useful. Treat for osteoporosis.

BIPOLAR DISORDER (mania/manic depression): is one of those descriptive diagnosis that "orthodox" psychiatry issues. We would estimate that as many as 90% of the non-drug dependent patients are totally "curable" at home with home testing and home remedies. Food allergies, environmental sensitivities, hypoglycemia and hyperglycemia are the major considerations.

Testing for allergies can be accomplished using the pulse test and/or the diet diary and rotation elimination diet; the environmental sensitivities can be identified by the pulse test and avoidance/challenge tests; hypoglycemia and hyperglycemia require a six-hour GGT (be sure to record the emotions and behavior of the patient during the entire six hours — the numbers alone are not revealing in of themselves).

Foods that are common offenders are cow's milk, corn wheat, soy, rye and sugar; environmental culprits include house dust, perfume, formaldehyde and makeup; on the glucose tolerance test the mania and/or depression may occur on the ascending or the descending arms of the curve so someone must stay with the patients and record emotions and events!!!

Treatment of bipolar disorder requires a considerable effort on the part of the "doctor" and "nurse" because a positive turn around may take some weeks with temporary relapses.

Treatment should include chromium and vanadium at 500 mcg q.i.d.; autoimmune urine therapy for five to eight treatments; rotation or avoidance of offending foods; avoidance of sugar, caffeine, environmental allergens; essential fatty acids at 5 gm t.i.d.; niacin (B-3) 450 mg. q.i.d. in time release tablets; B-1, B-5, B-6 each at 100 mg b.i.d.; DL-phenylalanine at 5 gms b.i.d. and choline at 250 mg b.i.d. Plant derived colloidal minerals that contain lithium may be useful.

BIRTH DEFECTS: are a national crime in the United States! More than 98% are the result of preconception and early pregnancy malnutrition of the embryo! Today there are more teenagers that give birth to Down's Syndrome babies than women over 35. Cleft lips, cleft palates, hernias, heart defects, limb defects, spina bifida, etc are all examples of preventable diseases that have been eliminated by the veterinary profession by taking great pains to give proper nutrition to the female lab animal, pet and farm species before and during pregnancy — if you want to see why Americans have such a low rating when it comes to preventing birth defects (23rd in the world!!!) just go to a zoo on a Sunday or a fast food operation and watch what the teenage girls and pregnant women eat!

Prevention of birth defects requires more than "prenatal" vitamins after the second month of pregnancy when the "orthodox" doctor gives his pronouncement "you're pregnant" — by then the embryo has formed all organs and tissues (for better or worse!). Conscious attention to preconception vitamins and colloidal minerals and avoidance of alcohol is especially important to teenage and middle age mothers-to-be; don't wait for anyone's advice — it isn't going to come. Do a home pregnancy test as soon as you think you're pregnant — if you haven't been taking supplements, start immediately!!!

BLADDER STONES (kidney stones, cystic calculi): are ironically caused by a calcium and/or a magnesium deficient diet. The minerals in the "stones" come from your own bones!!! Diagnosis may require an x-ray (a flat "plate" of the abdomen) — don't forget the gonadal

shield!!! The signal to think "stones" is blood in the urine (use the urine test sticks) and pain or "colic" that gets worse in the bladder or kidney area. "Stones" are potentially very painful and may require Tylenol-3 or morphine to cope with the pain if they are obstructing a ureter (the tube from the kidney to the bladder).
Treatment should include an anti-inflammatory medication such as licorice (Glycyrrhiza glabra) to reduce swelling at the "log jam" so the "stones" can pass — if this isn't strong enough, you may have to take prednisone for three (3) days to accomplish this part of the therapy. Calcium and magnesium at 2,000 mg and 1,000 mg is imperative to stop calcium loss from the bones; reduce meat intake (go more toward the vegetarian scale) to get your dietary calcium/ phosphorus ratio in order; herbs including dandelion (Taraxacum officinale), khella (Ammi visnaga), madder tea (Rubia tinctorium) and rupturewort tea (Hernia glabra); unsweetened cranberry juice to acidify the urine.

BLEEDING: from superficial wounds is an easy medical problem to deal with by using pressure with a sterile gauze "sponge" or a "bandaid" on digits. Bleeding in the stool, on the other hand, can be a serious symptom indicating stomach ulcers (black blood stool), ulcerative colitis (bloody mucus in stool), colon cancer (bloody mucus in the stool); or coughing blood — lung cancer, etc.

Diagnosis of the serious causes of "bleeding" will require some sophisticated diagnostic techniques performed by a "user friendly" physician (depending on the state, this may include an N.D., D.C., D.O., or M.D.).
Regardless of the cause superficial bleeding may be treated with poultices of plantain (Plantago major). The

specific therapies for the more serious problems will be dealt with as they are discussed.

BLEEDING BOWELS: can be part of the irritable bowel syndrome, chronic diarrhea or intestinal catarrh, hemorrhoids can show bright red blood on the toilet paper after passing a stool — again on a serious note one needs to consider bowel cancer. Amoebic dysentery and other parasites should also be considered in the diagnosis.
Treatment for the bleeding bowel should include mullein (Verbascum thapsus), vitamin C at 1,000 mg t.i.d. as time release tablets, alfalfa and specific therapy per diagnosis.

BLEEDING GUMS: an early warning for several problems, including vitamin C deficiency (scurvy), calcium deficiency (or bad calcium/phosphorus ratio — osteoporosis), receding gums (the gums recede because of underlying bone loss) or vitamin E deficiency.
Treatment should include vitamin C to bowel tolerance, vitamin E at 800 IU/day, correct dietary calcium/ phosphorus ratio with supplemental calcium/magnesium at 2,000 mg and 800 mg, herbal therapy including mouthwash with alpine ragwort (Senecio fuchsii) and mouthwash with aloe/hydrogen peroxide.

BLOATING (gastric): is the accumulation of gas in the stomach. Normally the stomach is sterile because of the acid environment, however, when hypochlorhydria (low stomach acid) occurs bacteria from the small intestine migrates up into the stomach. The bacteria in the stomach now "ferments" carbohydrates and sugars that are eaten and produce gas or "bloat."
Treatment of "bloat, belch and burp" includes oral hydrogen peroxide (20 drops/ oz.) at 1 oz. b.i.d., colloidal

minerals and betaine HCl and pancreatic enzymes at 75-200 mg t.i.d. 15 minutes before meals.

BODY ODOR (foot odor): can occur in anyone, especially teenagers and older people.
Treatment includes zinc at 50 mg t.i.d., calcium/magnesium at 2,000 mg and 800 mg, plant derived colloidal minerals at 1 oz. per 100 pounds; lots of green leafy vegetables, alfalfa, and baths and deodorants with hydrogen peroxide.

BOILS (carbuncles, abscesses): are usually caused by a "staph" infection of the skin and hair follicles. Boils can occur at a site of irritation — usually the neck near a collar line. The tender pus filled "boil" can be brought to a "head" by poultices of 3% boric acid and opened with a blade.
Treatment includes flushing the boil with sand sagebrush (Artemisia fififolia), enchinacea (Echinaca angustifolia) and/or hydrogen peroxide; vitamin C at bowel tolerance, vitamin A at 300,000 IU/day as beta carotene, zinc 50 mg t.i.d.; antibiotic ointment may be considered if new boils appear until the vitamins and minerals begin to take effect (don't forget the base line supplements).

BONE PAIN (including "spurs"): can be immobilizing and crippling. Bone pain can be part of the "growing pains" especially at the joints or the insertions of tendons into bones (which is where "spurs" occur). Bone pain is a self-diagnosing problem — if it persists, x-rays should be taken to confirm diagnosis of fracture, arthritis, "spurs" or rule the more severe problem of primary or metastatic bone cancer.
Treatment of bone pain and "spurs" includes vitamin C to bowel tolerance, vitamin E at 800-1,200 IU/day; mag-

nesium at 500 mg t.i.d. for as long as one to two years; correct the calcium/phosphorus ratio with calcium at 2,000 mg/day, reduce meat intake; herbs including comfrey (Symphytum officinale). Plant derived colloidal minerals have reversed spurs and calcium deposits without surgery by remodeling the bone.

BREAST CYSTS (fibrocystic disease): is a painful and cosmetic disease yet benign. The normal breast tissue is overgrown with scar tissue and cyst formation (usually multiple cysts). Prevention is simple enough and is related to avoidance of methyl xanthines (i.e., caffeine, coffee, tea, chocolate, etc.).
Treatment includes elimination of methyl xanthines from the diet, essential fatty acids 5 gm t.i.d. and vitamin E at 800-1,200 IU per day.

BREAST TENDERNESS (PMS): is a common symptom of PMS and early pregnancy. The tenderness of PMS is cyclical and that of early pregnancy will be associated with missed periods and a positive home pregnancy test.

Treatment includes vitamin E topically and essential fatty acids orally at 5 gm t.i.d., avoid methyl xanthines and remember the base line supplements.

BRITTLE NAILS: are a common ailment, especially in teenagers pregnant women and individuals with food allergies. The causes of brittle nails are malabsorption or deficiencies of essential fatty acids, amino acids (low protein-vegetarian diets), calcium, iron or zinc.
Treatment of brittle nails includes dealing with food allergies (use the pulse test — it's cheap and accurate) to improve absorption, gelatin (unflavored and unsweetened or diabetic brands), essential fatty acids at 5 gm

t.i.d., vitamin E at 800-1,200 IU/day, the base line supplementation, and betaine HCl and pancreatic enzymes at 75-200 mg each t.i.d. 15 minutes before meals.

BRONCHIAL ASTHMA: (see asthma)

BRONCHITIS (grippe, catarrh, chest colds): can be caused by viral or bacterial infections. Allergies, both food and inhalant will aggravate bronchitis as will fatty acid deficiencies. If bronchitis persists after treatment for five to ten days, consider cystic fibrosis in children and lung cancer in adults (x-rays will be necessary to determine chronic processes).

Treatment includes steam vaporizers at night, essential fatty acids at 5 gm t.i.d., digestive enzymes and betaine HCl at 75-200 mg each, vitamin C to bowel tolerance, vitamin A at 300,000 IU as beta carotene, zinc at 50 mg t.i.d. and herbs including slippery elm (Ulmus fulva), coltsfoot (Tussilago farfara), cowslip (Primula veris), eucalyptus (Eucalyptus globulus) as a poultice/chest rub and/or place in vaporizer, Irish moss (Chondrus crispus), pansy (Viola tricolor), pleurisy root (Asclepias tuberose) and holly hock (Althaea rosea).

BRUISES: are the result of a bump or blow that ruptures blood vessels and releases blood into the surrounding tissue including the skin. The fragility (tenderness) or capillaries can result from vitamin C or vitamin E deficiencies.

Treatment includes vitamin C to bowel tolerance, vitamin E at 800-1,200 IU per day, pancreatic enzymes at 200 mg t.i.d. between meals (so the enzymes get into your bloodstream and dissolve blood clots), DMSO topically, pain gel and herbs including arnica (Arnica montana), marigold (Calendula officinalis), witch hazel (Hamaelis virginiana) and yellow sweet clover (Metilotus officinalis).

BRUXISM (teeth grinding): is the clenching or grinding of teeth. Bruxism usually occurs during sleep and is, therefore, often overlooked until wear of the dental enamel is observed. Bruxism can be the result of food allergies (use the pulse test to find out - milk and wheat tend to be the offenders), hypoglycemia (bed-wetting may occur with bruxism if hypoglycemia is involved) or deficiencies of calcium, magnesium and / or B-6.
Treatment includes avoidance or rotation of offending food and elimination of sugar from the diet especially before bed. Calcium and magnesium at 2,000 mg and 1,000 mg per day and B-6 at 50 mg t.i.d.

BURNS: are the painful result of contact with radiant (sun) or thermal heat (fire or hot materials). Prevention of sunburn is easy with modern "sun screen" products — the nose may need special protection of zinc oxide ointment.
1st degree - red, painful surface burns from "sunburn," steam, etc. Dilute white vinegar 1:1 with water and cover burn surface twice daily, aloe vera or vitamin E oil applied locally.
2nd degree - some degree of damage into the second layer of skin with blisters. Bath the burn area with vitamin E oil, colloidal silver or cover with zinc oxide. Supplementation of vitamin C to bowel tolerance will be of value.
3rd and 4th degree burns are characterized by loss of skin, blisters and, in the case of the 4th degree, actual charring takes place. These types of burns require professional help to prevent infection and fluid loss; the patient may require "plastic surgery."

BURSITIS: is an inflammation of bursal sacs that cushion tendons as they pass over joints (i.e., shoulder, "housemaid's knee," "miner's elbow," and "bunions"). Overwork of an "out-of-shape" joint can bring on a flare up. Don't forget the base line vitamins and minerals as a preventative along with moderate exercise.

Treatment of bursitis includes topical pain gels, DMSO, or liniments with eucalyptus to bring more circulation to the area and remove swelling (which is the source of bursitis pain). Oral support includes B-12 at 1,000 mcg/day, vitamin C to bowel tolerance, bioflavonoids 1,200 mg/day, rutin 50 mg t.i.d., vitamin E at 800-1,200 IU/day, calcium and magnesium at 2,000 mg and 1,000 mg per day respectively, gelatin, cartilage 5 gm t.i.d. and alfalfa. Be sure to include plant derived colloidal minerals in your bursitis program.

CALCULUS (tartar): is a build up of calcium carbonate on the tooth, usually at the gingival junction (where the gum attaches to the tooth. The source of the calcium is the patient's own bony calcium which is being lost in the saliva (that's why tartar is worst on the back of the lower incisors) — when this happens you may need more magnesium to hold calcium in the bones and correct a severe dietary calcium/ phosphorus ratio problem (i.e., reduce red meat, soft drinks and any other major source of phosphorus). The use of hydrogen peroxide tooth gels and antitartar toothpastes will help reduce existing tartar and prevent build up.

Treatment of tartar includes flossing, use a "dental pick" that you can purchase from a pharmacy to pop off large "plates" of hardened tartar from the back of and between teeth, use a firm toothbrush and hydrogen peroxide tooth gels and tartar control toothpaste. Treat for osteoporosis.

CANCER (carcinoma, sarcoma, neoplasm, tumor and malignancy): is one of the more formidable syndromes (a disease is "one diagnosis/one cause") of today. Prevention is the "magic bullet" that is effective against all forms of cancer.

Prevention of cancer (CA) takes a considerable conscious effort, but then, aren't you worth the same or more effort than the maintenance of your Porsche!!! Don't forget the base line vitamins and colloidal minerals, be sure to incorporate dietary fiber in each meal, try to OD on beta carotene (almost impossible — first sign is dry skin) at about a vitamin A equivalent of 300,000 IU per day, lowfat diet (don't forget the essential fatty acids for your immune system), eat four-six cups of vegetables each day, drink eight glasses of water per day (preferably filtered — distilled water on a regular basis will demineralize your bones!), don't smoke, alcohol in moderation (or better yet — not at all), make sure you have at least two bowel movements per day (better yet, three), use sunscreens in intense sunlight, take alfalfa daily in some form as a detox, do a liver flush once or twice each month, do a hair analysis each year to monitor toxic metal load as well as absorption capability (if you are not absorbing very well all your nutrient minerals will be low), check for food allergies, (use the pulse test), use biodegradable household cleaners, avoid foods fried in fat or oil and use organic foods as much as possible.

The diagnosis of cancer usually requires a biopsy, x-ray or the use of endoscopic exams; elevated CEA or PSA are signals to look farther. You are your own first line of defense, therefore, if you find an unusual lump, ulcer, bleeding, extended diarrhea, pain, change in urination or bowel habit or mole that changes character you should consider cancer as a possible cause. If you do suspect cancer, start with your own therapies right away; it may be weeks before you can get to the "orthodox" doctor for a "rule-in" or "rule-out" diagnosis — don't go for six months without treatment because the "doctor was too busy" — what's more important, your health or his golf game? Once cancer has been "ruled-in" you should intensify your efforts in your own behalf as no one cares as much about you as much as you do!!!

Treatment of cancer is a busy procedure at the best and until you get it "under control" it will take your full time whether you opt to take the "CUT, BURN & POISON" route as well or if you opt totally for alternative therapies. A useful fact to help your thinking process is that the United States government says that THE FIVE-YEAR SURVIVAL RATE OF CANCER PATIENTS HAS NOT CHANGED OVER THE LAST 20 YEARS DESPITE NEW TECHNIQUES IN SURGERY, RADIATION ANDCHEMOTHERAPY — IN FACT, UNTREATED PATIENTS, AS A GROUP, SURVIVED LONGER!!! What the government doesn't tell you is that the "untreated" patient group includes those treated with alternative therapies!!

As with any therapy, you will want to educate yourself to benefits and limits of alternative therapies. Using one system or medication for cancer therapy is like limiting the United States defense system to ground forces (this would be a totally absurd line of thinking in these days of nuclear warfare, ICBMs, submarines, etc.). Fortunately, other countries do not have an FDA and, as a result, they have more pharmaceutical companies willing to search for, and make available, medications that our FDA forbids. As a result, our health in terms of dollars spent (800 billion) and return places us 23rd in the world — kind of frightening, isn't it! A list of medications follow with a brief discussion of the action of each and for what cancer they are recommended (most can be administered to yourself on a maintenance level once the cancer is under control):

HYDRAZINE SULFATE: inhibits the production of glucose from lactic acid in the liver which literally starves the rapidly growing cancer cells. Hydrazine can prevent metastasis (spreading) and will reduce the size of large tumor masses. The shrinkage of tumor mass has all kinds of benefit including increase in appetite, feeling of well being, reduction in pain, mood improvement and an improvement in circulation (blood and lymph). This compound is nonspecific and can be used for any tumor type cancer.

CESIUM CHLORIDE: provides "high pH therapy for cancer" by entering the cancer cell and causing an alkaline environment. It is recommended for all types of cancer but is particularly effective for SARCOMA, BRONCHOGENIC CARCINOMA (with bone metastasis) and a spectacular 97% improvement of COLON CANCER.

LAETRILE: in short, releases small amounts of cyanide which normal cells can detoxify but cancer cells can't. The cyanide from the laetrile then kills the cancer cell. Laetrile may be taken as a preventative measure or a therapy.

GERMANIUM: is found in significant amounts in a variety of plants including mushrooms, ginseng, garlic, etc. Germanium functions by increasing the oxygen flow into cells from the blood (cancer cells do not like high levels of oxygen), increases macrophage (scavenger cells) activity, increases the numbers of antibody forming cells, T-cells, B-lymphocytes and killer cells and induces the body to produce interferon!!! Can be used as prevention or in therapy programs.

CLODRONATE: is especially useful for preventing and controlling bone metastasis (spread of cancer from original site to the bone) which is common place in BREAST and PROSTATIC CANCER. Bone metastasis are very painful and difficult to treat with conventional chemotherapy, clodronate works by stopping the loss of calcium from the bone so that the cancer can be effectively walled off.

FLUTAMIDE: and luteinizing hormone-releasing hormone (LHRH) together are more effective than surgical or chemical castration in cases of PROSTATIC CANCER as well as more aesthetically accepted. Flutamide therapy works well against the original cancer as well as the metastatic bone cancer. Flutamide produces an 81% remission against 0% remission for two years when compared with "orthodox" approaches.

HOXEY HERBAL FORMULA: is one of the granddaddies of the modern cancer remedies. It is nonspecific and may be used like Laetrile as a preventive or remedy.

LEVAMISOL: is a new product (actually a sheep wormer) that has shown excellent results for cancer in general and specifically for colon, breast, brain, throat, esophagus, stomach, liver and pancreas. LEVAMISOL could be the cancer "magic bullet" for the 1990s!!!

POLYERGA: inhibits tumor growth by reduction of glycolysis. Polyerga is effective against tumor forming cancer and can be easily administered at home — it is, therefore, very economical.

There are many adjunctive therapies for cancer programs (remember it is absurd to use single mode programs!) amongst which hydrogen peroxide stands out. "Orthodox" medicine used H_2O_2 IV in the 1800s so there is lots of history with no bad side effects as well as lots of positive evidence that increasing oxygen in the blood has beneficial effects in your fight against cancer (remember cancer doesn't like elevated oxygen levels).

CO Q-10 increases the immune fighting ability of your phagocytes as well as increases the efficiency of tissue detoxification.

DMSO is useful for the treatment of LEUKEMIA in that it causes the maturation of the "premature" WBCs of leukemia.

Thymus extracts are useful to enhance the thymus gland function and thus the immune system.

Autoimmune urine and autoimmune blood therapies enhance the bodies defense systems against foreign substances including cancer proteins in much the same way the "allergy shots" do against pollen allergies.

Carbamide (urea) is in keeping with the autoimmune urine therapy. Carbamide is particularly effective for LIVER CANCER.

Beta carotene taken with vitamin E can be taken at as much as 600,000 IU vitamin A equivalent!!! This will be of significant benefit in cancer therapy programs especially CARCINOMAS. The vitamin A thus provided will also help the thymus gland produce antibodies and make laetrile more effective.

Selenium is a trace mineral that has been investigated very intensively as a cancer preventative and as therapeutic nutrition, 1,000-3,000 mcg/day is considered to be the proper therapy dose. Plant derived colloidal selenium is 98% absorbable.

Shark cartilage and shark liver oil contain substances that stop the formation of capillaries that feed new metastatic growths of cancer.

Chemotherapy in "micro-doses" in conjunction with alternative therapies or chemotherapy into the arterial blood supply of the cancer infested tissue or organ can substantially reduce the negative side effects of chemotherapy.

Intravenous infusions with total nutrition, especially in the early phases of alternative therapy are very useful in providing your body with much needed raw material for rebuilding normal tissue as well as replenishing the ravaged immune system. This total nutrition should include vitamins, minerals amino acids, essential fatty acids as well as electrolytes. It is well established that cancer patients have poor digestion and absorption (probably from the long term effects of food allergies on the gut producing celiac type changes).

CANDIDIASIS (chronic fatigue syndrome): is an infection caused by Candida albicans, a normally harmless yeast (saprophyte) of your intestine. This organism becomes a parasite and, therefore, pathological (disease creating) when its competitors, the normal bacteria of the gut, are killed by long term use of antibiotics allowing them to proliferate unchecked. The reduced production of stomach acid allows the C. albicans to move into the stomach — an unusual location. Stress will cause the reduction of stomach acid after stress reaches the point of decompensation. Food allergies change the lining of the gut in a manner very similar to celiac disease which causes an increased nutrient concentration in the gut — this hyperfertilized environment is very attractive to C. albicans. The overgrowth of the organism eventually spills over into the blood stream and, thus, infests the body proper.

Prevention includes being aware of your intestines, know your digestive and absorptive abilities and patterns. Do pulse tests for food allergies, avoid long term use of antibiotics, as you grow older take betaine HCl and pancreatic enzymes before meals to offset the normal decrease in production (take these digestive aids if you are under stress), deal aggressively with any disease that lowers your immune capacity!

The diagnosis of candidiasis may be made from symptoms, however, if you want a sure diagnosis get a blood test for antibodies against C. albicans or a skin test (very similar to a TB tine test) — a positive test is a sure diagnosis — a negative test may or may not be revealing. Anergy is a state in which the immune system is so exhausted that it can't even react to a diagnostic test!!!

Symptoms of candidiasis include forgetfulness, irritability, fatigue, nausea, flu-like joint and muscle pain and a high emotional state. Gastrointestinal symptoms may or may not be present (i.e., diarrhea, dyspepsia, gas, etc.). Most of the patients we see have been on oral Nystatin for some length of time with little or no positive effect — no wonder, Nystatin is not absorbed into the body proper and, therefore, only controls the C. albicans in the gut.

Treatment for candidiasis includes treating food allergies, hypoglycemia, any concurrent infection (i.e., herpes, EBV, CMV, etc.) and correcting indigestion. Hydrogen peroxide may be taken orally at 1 oz. b.i.d. upon arising and retiring (we like H_2O_2 that is mixed with aloe vera which makes it palatable and makes it easy to take (also there is no danger in this diluted form). Hydrogen peroxide in a DMSO and 5% dextrose solution should be administered IV to kill the systemic infestation (it takes 10-12 infusions to get the desired effect).

Germanium orally and IM is a good adjunctive therapy as it helps get oxygen into the cells (remember C. albicans doesn't like oxygen) making the general environment unattractive to the parasite.
Replantation of Lactobacillus acidophilus, a friendly resident of the gut and a primary competitor to C. albicans is a useful part of any treatment program. Using the retention enemas with 4 oz. of warm water containing 10 billion organisms (empty twenty 500,000 organism capsules into the water). A retention douche of 3 oz. for ten minutes weekly. The external genital area in both male and female may be washed with 3% hydrogen peroxide. Sixteen ounces of 3% hydrogen peroxide can safely be added to bath water. Autoimmune urine and blood therapies can be very useful in stimulating specific antibody production.

CANKER SORES (cold sores, fever blisters, aphthous stoma-stomatitis): can be precipitated by stress, consumption of certain foods as in food allergies (do the pulse test) and certain deficiencies. The canker sore is differentiated from Herpes in that it only occurs on the movable oral mucosa of the lips and cheeks.
Treatment should include avoidance of allergens, zinc at 50 mg t.i.d., lysine at 1,500 mg/day, vitamin E at 800-1,200 IU/day, B-complex at 50 mg each t.i.d. and vitamin A at 300,000 IU/day as beta carotene.

CARBUNCLES (multiple boils): See BOILS

CARDIAC ARRHYTHMIA (irregular heart beat): is a common complaint of persons with food allergies and hypoglycemia (this is assuming you have ruled out organic heart disease). The classic for this syndrome is the "Chinese restaurant syndrome" which is caused by sensitivity to MSG. Many a patient with sudden irregular heart beat and palpitations has called the ambulance thinking they had a "heart attack;" by the time the ambulance arrived, they no longer had symptoms — a history of eating out, especially at a Chinese restaurant, is the give away.

Deficiencies that cause cardiac arrhythmia include B-1 (i.e., beriberi), B-3 (i.e., pellagra), B-6, chromium, Selenium (i.e., Keshan Disease, cystic fibrosis), magnesium, potassium, carnitine and CO Q-10.

Treatment of cardiac arrythmia includes avoidance of known allergens, autoimmune urine and blood therapies, chromium at 50-100 mcg t.i.d., B-complex at 50 mg t.i.d., selenium at 100-300 mcg t.i.d., magnesium at 1,000 mg/day, potassium at 500 mg t.i.d., plant derived colloidal minerals, carnitine and CO Q-10 per label.

CARDIOMYOPATHY (Keshan Disease, muscular dystrophy of heart): is recognized by the WHO as a selenium deficiency. This is the type of heart disease that makes individuals a candidate for heart transplant in the eyes of the "orthodox" physician. It is typical that $1/month in selenium supplement would prevent this disease and the "need" for a $250,000 procedure that carries a 20% mortality rate. This disease is also found in cystic fibrosis patients (one of the telltale signals that genetics has nothing to do with cystic fibrosis). Cardiomyopathy is known as "mulberry heart disease" in pigs and "white muscle disease" in cattle, sheep and horses — it is interesting that veterinarians have eliminated this disease in animals with selenium injections and oral supplementation of diets (again an example where it just might be better to go to your vet!!!).

The diagnosis of cardiomyopathy is made from an ECG

(electrocardiogram) in an "orthodox" cardiologists office. The earliest signs are S-T and T wave changes — at this point, diet correction and selenium supplementation will reverse this if the diagnosis is correct — the neglect of this will result in severe fatigue and sufficient heart muscle changes for the cardiologist to be able to "justify" a heart transplant.

The treatment of early cardiomyopathy includes selenium at 350 mcg t.i.d. or 1,000 mcg IM, plant derived colloidal selenium, vitamin E at 1,200 IU/day and essential fatty acids at 5 gm t.i.d. I have personally seen individuals who have survived quite well with only selenium supplementation — they still have mild S-T or T wave changes but they have been working out in the rice fields for 25 years after their diagnosis and treatment with selenium!!!

CARPAL TUNNEL SYNDROME (SLIPPED TENDION PEROSIS): is caused by compression of the median nerve in between the tendons of the forearm muscles by a shrinking of the circular wrist ligament that holds everything together. This compressed nerve causes radiating pain in the palm of the hand and wrist, especially when the underside of the wrist is forcefully tapped with an index finger or a reflex hammer. Carpal tunnel syndrome is caused by a deficiency of arsenic, manganese and choline.

Treatment includes B-6 at 75 mg t.i.d., zinc at 50 mg t.i.d., plant derived colloidal arsenic, manganese and choline (compare this with the "orthodox" therapy of wrist surgery!!!).

CARSICKNESS (sea sick, air sick): or motion sickness is common in some individuals when repetitive angular and linear movement occur at the same time. Fixing the gaze on a single geographic point can help in sea sickness when the patient is on deck but a fruitless exercise in other forms of motion sickness. Symptoms include "green at the gills" feeling including nausea and vomiting.

Prevention of motion sickness includes the use of scopolamine transdermal patches (can be worn behind the ear) or Dramamine (both medications can be purchased at the pharmacy without a prescription).

CATARACTS: are caused by changes in the eye lens which makes them opaque and unable to transmit light to the retina of the eye. Cataracts are easily diagnosed with the ophthalmoscope in a darkened examining room — severe cataracts are snow white and are easily seen with the unaided eye. Cataracts are the most common cause of blindness in older people and should be dealt with aggressively and without delay.

Treatment of cataracts includes the base line vitamin/mineral supplement plus vitamin E at 400 IU/day, vitamin C to bowel tolerance, B-1, B-2, B-3, B-5 and B-6 at 50 mg b.i.d., inositol at 150 mg/day, selenium at 250 mcg/day, zinc at 25 mg t.i.d., bioflavonoids at 300 mg, glycine at 200 mg, 1-glutamine at 200 mg, 1-arginine at 300 mg/day, l-cysteine at 400 mg/day and glutathione at 40 mg/day. If diabetes or hypoglycemia are present the chromium at 50 mcg t.i.d. should be added.

CATARRH (croup, whooping cough): is the mucus associated with a wide variety of nasal, throat, tracheal and bronchial infections and/or irritations.

Treatment includes the use of steam at bedtime to break up the catarrh (mucus) and allow peaceful sleep, if this does not work and sleep in an urgent need the use of drying agents such as Contac should be considered. Homeopathy can work quite well if a complete case is collected (see homeopathy) as there are many variables to be considered. Herbs that can be effective include vervain or wild hyssop (Verbena officinalis), cucumber (Cucumis sativa), wild cherry (Prunis serotina) and thyme (Thymus vulgaris).

CELIAC DISEASE (gluten enteropathy, nontropical spruce): is perhaps the most underrated disease in America today. Celiac disease is characterized by a loss of villi (finger-like projections) from the small intestines and a scaring of the supporting tissue which effectively reduces the absorptive surface by 70%. Classically celiac disease is caused by a wheat gluten sensitivity, thus "gluten free diets" — if this change was limited to wheat only, it would be of small consequence because it is easily recognized, however, cow's milk albumen and soy protein will cause these same physical changes in the gut including loss of villi and scaring of supportive tissue of the small intestine progressing to the point where by age 45-50 years, 90% of the intestine can be damaged resulting in a significant reduction of absorptive surface. The result is poor assimilation of nutrients which are the raw materials for tissue repair, growth and maintenance of the immune system.

Celiac disease is, therefore, the basic cause of many diseases including diabetes (i.e., malabsorption of chromium and vanadium), cancer (i.e., malabsorption of zinc, vitamin A and selenium), and muscular dystrophy and cystic fibrosis (i.e., malabsorption of selenium in the pregnant mother resulting in damage to the fetus).

Diagnosis and treatment of celiac disease includes using the pulse test for allergies (i.e., whole wheat is great unless your allergic to it!!!) especially wheat, cow's milk and soy products and eliminating and/or rotating the offending allergen — it takes 90 days to repair the injured gut which means there is great hope if you take the effort to see if, in fact, you are sensitive to wheat, cow's milk or soy.

CEREBROPALSY: is a birth defect which affects the cerebellum, the fine motor coordinator of the body. The cause is a preconception deficiency of zinc and B-6 (perhaps celiac disease was the base cause of copper / zinc malabsorption in the mother). There is no treatment since the damage occurred to the fetus during the formation of the brain.

CEREBROVASCULAR DISEASE (senile dementia): is more common in the United States than anywhere else. The "hardening" of the middle cerebral artery (the main blood supply to the brain) results in poor oxygen supply to the brain which causes loss of memory and typical "senile" changes. As with arteriosclerosis, the "hardening" of the arteries is caused by smooth muscle scaring, followed by calcification and fatty cholesterol deposits. The risk factors include elevated blood cholesterol which is a building block of vitamin D — vitamin D is angiotoxic (toxic to blood vessels) causing scaring of arterial smooth muscle and subsequent calcification. Magnesium deficiency also results in calcification.
Prevention includes comfortable collars and ties so "eddies" are not created in the carotid arteries which contributes to the deposition of cholesterol. Reduce the amount of vitamin D intake to a maximum of 400 IU/day (this is a real toughie when you consider animal fat, cholesterol, milk, butter, various prepared cereals and snack bars, supplements and sunshine).

Treatment of cerebrovascular disease includes EDTA chelation therapy to help remove plaque, hydrogen peroxide IV to increase oxygen, vitamin C to bowel tolerance, avoid alcohol, vitamin E at 800-1,200 IU/day, essential fatty acids at 5 mg t.i.d., selenium at 1,000 mcg/day, centrophenoxine at 1,000-2,000 mg/day, hydergine at 4.5-9.0 mg/day, vasopressin (DIAPID) at 12-16 units/day, Lucidril at 4.4-8.0 gm/day, piracetam at 1.6 gm t.i.d. and choline at 9 gm/day concurrently, and lecithin at 4 gm b.i.d.

CERVICAL DYSPLASIA: is considered a "precancerous" change in the surface cells of the uterine cervix. The "orthodox" approach, cryotherapy, is primarily a "counter-irritant" procedure — in other words, create enough acute damage so that the influx of WBCs and antibodies also help heal chronic changes as a "side benefit." It is known that cervical dysplasia is, in fact, a manifestation of a chronic vitamin A deficiency. Diagnosis is made from a PAP smear and/or biopsy.

Treatment of cervical dysplasia is accomplished by painting the affected surface with Lugol's Solution (an iodine preparation) and oral supplementation of beta carotene at an equivalent of 300,000 IU of vitamin A per day and oral zinc at 50 mg t.i.d. Don't forget the base line nutritional supplement here.

CHALAZION: is the result of plugged "meibomian" glands in the eyelid. A chalazion is easily confused with a "sty" in the early stages, however, after a few days the swelling and pain disappear leaving a slow growing pea sized "mass" in the lid.

Treatment of chalazions include vitamin A at 300,000 IU per day as beta carotene, zinc at 50 mg t.i.d. and warm poultices of 3% boric acid on the closed lid. Boric acid ophthalmic ointment may be obtained from the pharmacy without prescription.

CHEILOSIS (angular stomatitis): is the result of vitamin B-2 or riboflavin deficiency. The deficiency shows upas cracks in the corners of the mouth, nasolabial folds and "geographic" tongue.
Treatment of cheilosis includes identification of food allergies and supplementation with B-2 at 75 mg t.i.d.

CHICKEN POX (Varicella, Herpes zoster-shingles): is an acute viral disease in children and a chronic, painful disease in adults (i.e., shingles). Epidemics occur in children in winter and early spring. Day care children are almost guaranteed to contract chicken pox in their first year of day care. For those that are into vaccination, a post exposure vaccine is available for up to 72 hours post exposure. Chicken pox is characterized by clear vesicles surrounded by a small red zone; these lesions occur primarily on the upper torso.
Treatment of chicken pox in children is primarily symptomatic and includes Caladryl lotion topically, oatmeal baths and vitamin E oil applied directly to each vesicle or papule. Regardless of therapy, chicken pox will last from seven to twenty days.

CHIGGERS (mites): are small arthropods (eight-legged critters) that burrow into the skin and cause a severe pruritis (itching). These little creatures can be repelled while walking in the woods or meadows by placing pet "flea collars" around your ankles, waist and wrists. The use of poultry dusting power can be used in socks or belt line.
Treatment of chiggers once they establish themselves is limited to covering each burrow opening with clear nail

polish which literally smothers them.

CHILLS (fever): are associated with the flu and other viral infections. The patient will be sweating, shaking, trembling and unable to feel warm even when bundled up with blankets.
Treatment for chills includes wearing warmups with a hooded sweatshirt to cover the neck and head, homeopathy, acupuncture and herbs to include willow (Salix alba).

CHILBLAINS (hypothermia): is the lowering of body and/or limb temperature to subnormal levels for some length of time resulting in near frostbite. Severe numbness and loss of function may occur. Colds and flu may follow this challenge to the immune system. Prevention includes proper dress for the weather.
Treatment includes rapid warming in warm water and/or warm enemas, electric blankets if available (underneath as well as on top).

CHOLESTEROL (elevated): is considered a risk factor for cardiovascular disease. Elevation of cholesterol above 270 mg per 100 ml of blood is a sign of increasing risk for cardiovascular disease, diabetes and liver disease (including gallstones). There are numerous causes of elevated cholesterol including low fiber diets, elevated vitamin D intake, deficiency of EFA, chromium and vanadium, diets high in refined sugar and flour, liver malfunction and poor exercise habits. CAUTION: Low cholesterol can be equally or more dangerous than elevated cholesterol!
Treatment for elevated cholesterol includes regular exercise, base line supplement program, one to two heaping tablespoons of oat bran or protein fiber in an eight

oz. glass of juice or vitamin C to bowel tolerance, essential fatty acids at 5 gm t.i.d., niacin at 450 mg b.i.d. as time release tablets, calcium and magnesium at 2,000 mg and 1,000 mg per day, chromium at 75 mcg t.i.d., vanadium, selenium at 100 mcg t.i.d. and herbs to include evening primrose (Oenothera biennis). A good liver flush can be very useful.

CHOREA: is characterized by uncontrolled jerky or crampy type movements that may be regular in frequency. The onset of chorea is subtle and may be limited to mood changes, faltering or hesitant speech then progressing to uncontrolled facial movements and grimaces, "prancing" gait, torticollis (marked twist in the neck) and difficulty in swallowing. Chorea is considered to be a genetic disease by the "orthodox" doctors, however, this is highly unlikely as the onset classically occurs between the ages of 30 to 55 years (we have seen chorea in preteens and teenagers). There is organic disease of the brain with degeneration of the frontal cerebral cortex as well as deeper portions of the brain. The "orthodox" treatment for chorea is limited to sedation and tranquilization.

We recommend the base line supplement program, essential fatty acids at 5 gm t.i.d., B-complex at 100 mg b.i.d. each, vitamin E at 800-12,000 IU/day, selenium at 500 mg/day, lecithin at 2,500 mg t.i.d. and choline at 500 mg/day. Pulse testing for food allergies and hair analysis to monitor absorption is essential.

CHRONIC FATIGUE (candidiasis, EBV, HBLV, CMV, food allergies and hypoglycemia): by its very name (syndrome rather than a disease) lets you know that this is a complex of symptoms with multiple causal factors. To our knowledge all patients with Chronic Fatigue Syndrome have two or more of the causal factors associated with their "disease." Symptoms include moodiness, highly emotional state, aches, pains, depression, gastrointestinal symptoms (i.e., "belch, burp and bloat"), intense fatigue, drowsiness and muscular weakness. Blood tests for antibodies against Candida albicans, EBV, HBLV and CMV are available for specific diagnosis; there is also a skin test for candidiasis.

Treatment for Chronic Fatigue Syndrome should include IV hydrogen peroxide in a solution of DMSO and 5% dextrose, IV nutrition, IM germanium, base line nutritional supplement program, hydrogen peroxide (20 drops per oz. in aloe juice) 1 oz. b.i.d., do pulse test for food allergies, do six-hour GTT for hypoglycemia, eliminate caffeine, eliminate refined sugar, avoid any food allergens, treat hypoglycemia with chromium at 75 to 200 mg t.i.d., employ autoimmune urine and blood therapies, detoxify with liver flushes and colonics (especially for the first two weeks of therapy) to copy with toxins generated by organism die-off, Isoprinosin at 500 mg t.i.d. and Ribavirin at 250-1,200 mg per day as antiviral medication. Reflexology, massage and naturopathic or chiropractic manipulation are great adjunctive therapies.

CLAUDICATION (intermittent): is a cramping of leg muscles following exercise as a result of poor blood supply. The reduced blood supply to the legs is almost always due to arteriosclerosis of the femoral and popliteal arteries. Typically, after a few moments rest, the patient can start walking again.

The diagnosis of intermittent claudication can be made from symptoms alone; the symptomatic findings can be supported by taking the "pedal" pulses (at the instep of the foot); these pulses should be strong and equal — very frequently one or both are weak or absent.

Treatment of intermittent claudication includes the base line nutritional supplements, EDTA chelation therapy, IV hydrogen peroxide, vitamin C to bowel tolerance, vitamin E at 800-1,200 IU per day, chromium at 75-200 mcg t.i.d., selenium at 100-500 mcg t.i.d., B-6 at 100 mg b.i.d., hydrotherapy, reflexology, massage and light exercise (i.e., walking, swimming, etc.) and herbs including ginseng (Panax spp.) and cayenne pepper (Capsicum minimum).

CLIMACTERIC (menopause): is the cessation of ovarian function and the stopping of the menstrual cycle. Menopause is a natural event in a woman's life and usually occurs between the ages of 45-55 years. Menopause may be artificially induced by ovariectomy or hysterectomy. When the process is normal and thus takes a gradual course, the adrenals and liver increase their output of female hormones (primarily estrogen) and make up the difference from the lost ovarian function. "Hot flashes" are a common symptom when insufficient estrogen is being produced by the adrenals or liver. Other symptoms include sweating, nervousness, fatigue, depression, insomnia, tingling and urinary frequency and in continuance. Osteoporosis is a common result of improperly managed menopause.

Treatment for menopause is probably an improper term as normal events don't need treatment but rather "support" on occasion to help smooth the transition. Estrogen supplements should not be used as they increase the cancer induction risk; eat two eggs everyday; red meat once each day; liver flush at least once per month, base line supplement program, calcium and magnesium at 2,000 mg and 1,000 mg per day and herbs to include Lady's mantle (Alchemilla vulgaris), motherwort (Leo nurus cardiaca) and St. John's wort (Hypericum perforatum). Don't forget calcium and magnesium at 2,000 mg and 1,000 mg per day. Betaine HCl and pancreatic enzymes at 75-200 mg t.i.d. 15 minutes before meals.

"CLUSTER HEADACHES" (histamine headache): are related to allergic reactions and may occur by themselves or by associated with other diseases and syndromes including Chronic Fatigue Syndrome. The symptom of one sided headache that comes on suddenly, cause debilitating pain and come and go in severity is diagnostic. Pulse testing and rotation elimination diets with the use of a "diet diary" for keeping track of symptoms (in this case, the "cluster headache"). In addition to foods, there are many inhalant allergens including cigarette smoke, perfume, house dust, etc. that can precipitate "cluster headache."

Treatment includes the use of the base line supplement program, vitamin C to bowel tolerance, bioflavonoids at 150 mg t.i.d., autoimmune urine and blood therapy and avoidance of environmental allergens, avoidance or rotation of food allergens.

COLDS (nasal catarrh, coryza): are caused by more than 100 different viruses; this is why no vaccine has been made available. Symptoms last for 7-14 days regardless of therapy. The incubation is very short (1-3 days) compared to most viral infections (10-21 days) with a sudden appearance of symptoms which include tingling in nose and throat, scratchy throat, nasal mucus, coughing, headache and laryngitis. Elevated temperature or fever is variable depending on the particular virus that is causing the "cold."

Treatment of the "common cold" should include vitamin C to bowel tolerance, bioflavonoids at 150 mg t.i.d., garlic gelatin capsules at 10 mg t.i.d., base line supplement program, chicken rice soup (proven by Harvard to be "best cold therapy") for protein (to replace that lost in the mucus — yes, mucus is protein similar to egg white) and electrolytes (especially potassium), bed rest, avoid chills, homeopathy, herbs to include oldman's beard (Usnea barbata), bigleaf linden (Tilia platyphyllos), dogrose (Rosa canina), European elder (Sambucus nigra), European Holly (Ilex aquifolium), hemp acrimony (Eupatorium cannabinum), purple coneflower (Echinacea angustifolia), Queen-of-the-meadow (Filipendula ulmaria), sea buckthorn (Hippophae rhamnoides), white willow (Salix alba), wormwood (Artemisia absinthium), yellowbark cinchona or Peruvian bark (Cinchona succiruba), feverfew (Chrysanthemum parthenium), bachelor's buttons (Pyrethrum parthenium), sweet balm (Melissa officinalis) and cayenne pepper (Capsicum minimum).

COLIC (severe belly pain): can be initiated by a variety of causes including food allergies, hypochlorhydria (low stomach acid), gas bubbles from fermentation, to more serious causes such as kidney or gallstones or blocked bowel. In this section, we will limit the discussion to food allergies, hypochlorhydria and fermentation since they are all three related. Food allergies cause "celiac" like changes in the gut resulting in malabsorption; bowel organisms "ferment" the unabsorbed nutrients causing "bubbles" which cause sufficiently sharp pain from distension to create "colic" — this is especially true in babies. In adults, stress and/or food allergies can cause hypochlorhydria allowing organisms to move into the normally sterile stomach and ferment food crating the "belch, burp and bloat" syndrome or "colic."

The treatment for colic in adults includes the base line supplement program, betaine hydrochloride and pancreatic enzymes at 75-200 mg each t.i.d. 15 minutes before meals, pulse testing to determine presence of food allergies. In babies, pulse testing and diet diaries to determine offending foods, pancreatic enzymes at 75-200 mg t.i.d. before meals (enzymes may be constipating), one to two drops of flaxseed oil after each meal and B-6 at 10 mg b.i.d. In older children and adults herbs including dill (Peucedanum graveolens) may be of value.

COLITIS: is an inflammation of the colon which can be caused by stress, food allergies, bacterial or viral infections, low fiber diets, etc. Symptoms vary from cramping and diarrhea to constipation alternating with diarrhea, bloody mucus, ulcerative colitis and diverticulitis. Treatment includes cathartics or antidiarrheals as necessary, high fiber meals (i.e., potato, well cooked oat bran, multi-grain breads); do avoid raw carrots, peanuts and corn for the first week of therapy, use pulse test to determine if food allergies are involved — if so, use rotation diet and autoimmune urine and blood therapy, drink a minimum of eight glasses of water each day as well as four to six cups full of green leafy vegetables (i.e., spinach, cabbage, etc.) preferably steamed or cooked at the start of therapy, oral hydrogen peroxide (as SuperOxy Plus) 1 oz. b.i.d. and aloe powder (Aloe vera) at 65-300 mg per day.

CONGESTED LUNGS (with bronchitis): can be treated with homeopathy, acupuncture, hydrotherapy to include a steam sauna, massage, and herbs including penny royal (Mentha pulegium) as concentrated tea.

CONGESTIVE HEART FAILURE: can be caused by lung disease, high blood pressure, nutritional deficiencies including B-1 and selenium. There is usually a rapid irregular heart beat and edema (swelling from tissue water) in the legs and/or belly cavity ("dropsy"). Two medications stand out in their efficacy (these herbs are even used by the "orthodox" doctors): 1) Lily of the valley (Convallaria megalis) and 2) foxglove (Digitalis purpura). These two herbs can be taken as whole leaf preparations or fluid extracts (foxglove is potentially dangerous so you should get commercially prepared sources and advice on doses). English hawthorne (Crataegus oxyacantha) is a useful herb for regulating heart rhythm and treating dropsy of congestive heart failure, however, may not be strong enough in severe or advanced cases. The precipitating cause of the congestive heart failure should be identified and dealt with aggressively.

CONJUNCTIVITIS: is an inflammation of the membrane that forms the inner surface of the eyelids and covers the white of the eye. Dust, allergens (i.e., pollens), foreign bodies including eyelashes and microorganisms (bacteria and viruses) can all initiate conjunctivitis.
Treatment of conjunctivitis includes using commercial eye washes (hydrogen peroxide eye drops) and/or boric acid ophthalmic ointment as appropriate. Pulling the upper lid over the lower lid by grasping the eyelash, lifting out, then down induces tear flow to wash eye and flush foreign bodies.

CONSTIPATION: is not only uncomfortable put a significant risk factor for cancer. If you are not having two to three bowel movements per day, you are constipated!!! Very frequently exercise such as walking and eight glasses of water per day will solve simple constipation. Very frequently food allergies will initiate constipation (do pulse test to determine this factor). Milk products, including cheese has a constipating affect on certain individuals.

Treatment of constipation includes eight to ten glasses of water per day, fiber/protein at 1 tbsp. in 8 oz. of juice b.i.d., rotation/elimination diet and autoimmune urine therapy for allergies, four to six cups of vegetables per day, exercise for 30 minutes per day, homeopathy and herbs including castor oil (Rincinus communis), olive oil (Olea europaea), blackroot F (Leptondra virginica), American mandrake (Podophyllum peltatum), alder buckthorn (Rhamnus frangula), cascara sagrada (Rhamnus purshiana), flaxseed or oil (Linum usitatissimum), senna (Cassia angustifolia) and psyllium (Plantago psyllium).

CONTRACEPTION: is historically a touchy subject!! For knowledge of contraception and abortion herbs midwives were deemed to be "witches" and burned at the stake! Today, because of population problems, AIDS and teen pregnancies contraception cannot be ignored if we are to survive. Some governments have imposed "one child" limits on their citizens, give free contraceptives to anyone who asks for them and most are offering a form of "sex education." Sex outside of marriage is "Russian Roulette," anal sex is putting a loaded gun to your mouth and pulling the trigger!!!

Contraception is divided into abstinence, barriers, hormones (this is the least desirable from the standpoint of side effects), IUDs (intrauterine devices — be careful here — remember the Delcon Shield!!!), and surgery (vasectomy or tying the fallopian tubes). The "rhythm" method cannot be considered a safe form of contraception outside of the marriage because of the AIDS risk and few couples have the consistent self-control necessary to prevent pregnancies.

CONVULSIONS (seizures, fits): are uncontrolled body movements set off by an electrical malfunction of the brain. High "fevers" of 104.0-105.0 F are often a cause of convulsions in children. Epilepsy is a form of convulsion that is easily diagnosed by abnormal brain waves seen on an EEG (electroencephalogram). Unfortunately, the "orthodox" neurologist doesn't think "allergy" when a hysterical mother brings a child to his office with a history of one or more convulsions. The "orthodox" approach to treating convulsions is Dilantin and/or phenobarbital.

Treatment of non-temperature induced convulsions can include a pulse test to determine if allergies are a factor. If it is determined that allergies are associated with the convulsions the patient may avoid the foods or chemicals, rotate foods on a five-day "rotation" diet and take autoimmune urine therapy; take autoimmune urine therapy; high fat, high cholesterol diet; supplements of value include calcium and magnesium at 2,000 and 1,000 mg, B-6 at 100 mg b.i.d., chromium at 75-100 mcg t.i.d. and herbs to include peony (Paeonia officinalia), catnip (Nepeta cataria) and skullcap (Scutellaria lateriflora). Chiropractic and acupuncture can be of great value here.

COR PULMONALE: is classically thought of as an enlargement of the right ventricle of the heart as a result of severe and chronic lung disease (i.e., asthma, cystic fibrosis, bronchiectasis). There is usually a rapid pulse, palpitations and edema of head, neck and lungs (the latter can be fatal) and sometimes there is angina. "Clubbing" of the finger and toenails and cyanotic (blue from lack of oxygen) nail beds is frequently seen when the lung disease is chronic. X-ray will easily diagnose this

problem.
Treatment of cor pulmonale includes resolving the precipitating lung disease and oxygen, IV hydrogen peroxide and selenium at 500-1,000 mcg per day.

COUGHS (catarrh, asthma, chest complaints): are very bothersome and distracting to everyone around the patient. Coughs can be caused by minor irritations of the throat including allergies (i.e., milk), viral infections and chemical irritations. If a fever is present don't rule out milk allergies as milk allergies will cause a rise in temperature — use the pulse test!!!
Treatment should include avoidance of any allergen or irritant, autoimmune urine therapy (if allergic), steam vaporizers at night for sleep, and herbs to include anise (Pimpinella anismum), English plantain (Plantago lanceolata), licorice (Glycyrrhizaglabra), mullein (Verbascum densi-florum), thyme (Thymus vulgaris), onion (Alliumcepa), sweet chestnut (Castanea vesca) and comfrey (Symphytum officinale).

"CRABS" (pubic lice): are transmitted primarily by sexual contact. The "crab" (Phthirus pubis) causes a great deal of pubic and anal itching; they are relatively large yet difficult to see. Very close inspection with good lighting is required to find these insects. Very frequently dark "specks" of droppings of the lice can be found in white underwear.
Treatment should include specially formulated shampoos containing 1% gamma benzene hexachloride and direct removal of any visual "crabs."

"CRADLE CAP" (seborrheic dermatitis of infants): can occur as early as one month of age in babies. Cradle cap appears as a greasy thick crust on the scalp, behind the ears and face.

Treatment of cradle cap includes shampooing regularly to loosen the greasy scale, B-6 at 10-25 mg per day and zinc at 15-25 mg per day. Food allergies can contribute to this problem — do a pulse test.

CROHN'S DISEASE (regional enteritis): is a chronic infiltration or invasion of defensive WBCs and "macropohages" (special scavenger cells) into the terminal ileum (last portion of small intestine that joins with the colon). Several theories are currently in vogue as to the cause of Crohn's Disease including infection with T.B-like organisms (similar to Johne's Disease in camels!!!); of interest here is the high incidence of Crohn's Disease in Minnesota compared with all other areas of the United States. A second and perhaps more realistic cause is a food allergy (i.e., wheat, milk), do a pulse test and practice rigorous avoidance program of any identified allergens — this will prevent acute (sudden) attacks and actually result in reversal of the Crohn's changes to normal. Compare this with cortisone and surgery that the "orthodox" medics would have you choose!!!

Treatment of Crohn's Disease includes a high fiber diet (be sure to do a pulse test to be sure not to use the fiber you are allergic to!), folic acid at 5-10 mg t.i.d., vitamin A at 300,000 IU/day as beta carotene, B-12 at 1,000 mcg/day (best by injection in this disease), vitamin C to bowel tolerance if it can be tolerated. Calcium and magnesium at 2,000 and 1,000 mg per day (don't forget the base line supplement program here), selenium at 300 mcg t.i.d., chromium at 75 mcg t.i.d. and zinc at 50 mg t.i.d. Autoimmune urine therapy can be very useful.

CUTS (lacerations): are caused by paper, glass, metal,

knives and tools. Most cuts, except deep facial wounds, can be dealt with at home without "stitches" (sutures). Superficial cuts from kitchen knives, glass and metal can be cleaned with soap and water. The edges of the wound are then brought together with butterfly bandages or wound strips (Fig. 10-1). Actually there will be less scar formation with this method than with sutures.

Cuts contaminated with dirt (resulting from falls on gravel, concrete, wood or soil) need to be washed with soap and water to remove gross dirt and debris. The second step for contaminated wounds is to flush well with 3% hydrogen peroxide to "bubble" out the microscopic dirt that harbor microorganisms. The wound edges can then be brought together with butterfly bandages or wound strips, however, a drainage site should be provided (Fig. 10-2) to allow free exit to any possible infection. Bleeding from cuts can usually be stopped with pressure bandages unless an artery is cut. A cut artery will "spurt" blood each time the heart contracts. Small arteries can usually be controlled by pressure with a sterile sponge (gauze square), bleeding from a large artery in the arm or leg may require a tourniquet to control until you get professional help.

CYSTIC FIBROSIS (mucoviscidosis): is the "crime" of the century second only to diabetes (and that is only because diabetes affects millions and CF "only affects thousands each year") in that it is preventable, 100% curable in the early stages and can be far better managed in chronic cases than it is currently managed by "orthodox" medicine. Cystic fibrosis is an important fatal disease of humans. CF was originally thought to be limited to white populations of central European origin: today, CF has been diagnosed in all peoples of the earth.

CF is thought to be genetically transmitted by the "orthodox" pediatricians, yet "they" have failed to prove their theory despite multimillions of dollars spent in research. Classically, the diagnosis is made when any two of four criteria are present (Table 10-1), yet most "orthodox" pediatricians will not diagnose CF without a positive "sweat test" (elevated level of sodium, chloride and potassium in the sweat — greater than 65 mEq/L.

The "sweat test" has been elevated by dogma to "the diagnostic test" for CF yet there are at least 17 known diseases and syndromes that can give a positive sweat test (Table 10-2), leading at least one group of investigators to refer to CF as a syndrome rather than a disease. Initially described in 1933, CF was first thought to be the result of a vitamin A deficiency in children dying with celiac disease. In 1938, the term "cystic fibrosis" was coined because the pathologist mistakenly thought the changes in the pancreas were true cysts (fluid filled spaces lined with normal tissue). It is well known today that the "cysts" of CF are, in fact, a dilation of the pancreatic functional unit (acini) with atrophy (shrinking) of the lining tissue. In 1952, the fact that congenital CF occurred in a significant number of CF patients was established. The foundation of the genetic theory of CF transmission is based on the frequent congenital appearance and two very poor papers, one published in 1913 which claimed that two children with diarrhea had an "inborn error in fat metabolism" and one in 1965 that did an epidemiological study of a group of 232 Australian families with CF — despite six sets of twins, the study failed to shed clear light on the proposed genetic theory. These papers were so poor they would not get past the letter opener at any "orthodox" medical journal today. We have spent

Table 10-1. Four Criteria For The Diagnosis of Cystic Fibrosis

1. Exocrine Pancreatic Insufficiency
2. Bronchiectasis
3. Positive Sweat Test
4. Family History of the Disease

Table 10-2. Diseases and Symptoms That Have Reported Positive Sweat Test (1, 3, 9, 68, 72)

1. Adrenal Insufficiency
2. Ectodermal Dysplasia
3. Nephrogenic Diabetes Insipidus
4. Glucose-6 Phosphate Deficiency
5. Pupillatonia / Autonomic Dysfunction
6. Allergies
7. Calcifying Pancreatitis
8. Anorexia Nervosa
9. Cystic Fibrosis
10. Focal Hepatic Cirrhosis
11. Derangement of Prostaglandin Metabolism
12. Hypothyroidism
13. Fucosidosis
15. Malnutrition
16. Kwashiorkor
17. Diabetes

Figure 10-1. Butterfly Bandages for Clean Wounds

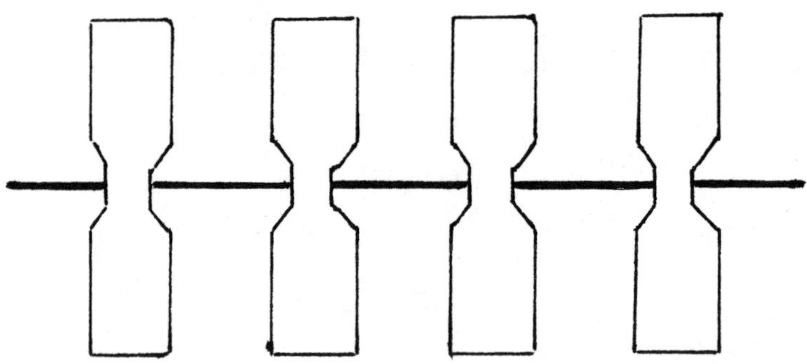

Figure 10-2. Butterfly Bandages for Contaminated Wounds

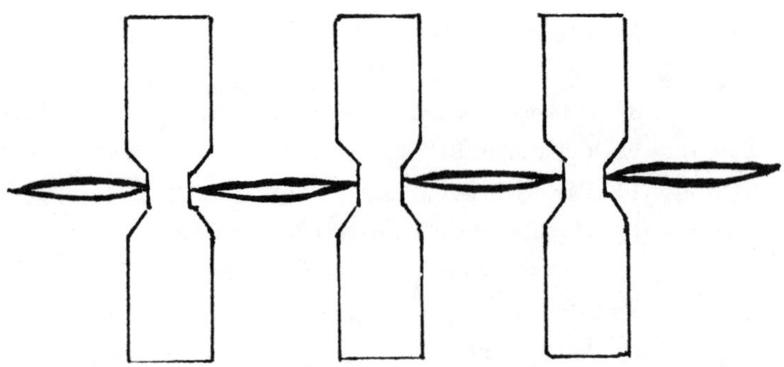

an inordinate amount of time on CF because this syndrome again demonstrates very clearly that if any medical specialty will be eliminated by discovery, that discovery will never be given to the public by the "orthodox" doctors!!!

In 1978, the first universally accepted diagnosis of CF in a laboratory animal was made by one of us (Dr. Joel Wallach). The diagnosis was based on characteristic CF changes in the pancreas and liver in baby monkeys and were confirmed by CF experts from Johns Hopkins School of Medicine, Emory University and the University of Chicago! Experts from NIH and the CF Foundation were overjoyed — that is until they learned that one of us (Wallach) could reproduce the CF changes with a congenital selenium deficiency in almost any animal species. With this revelation, Wallach was fired with 24 hours notice and "blackballed" from research (to show you how ruthless they are, Wallach was fired ten days after his wife died of cancer).

It has been learned recently that the positive "sweat test" is the result of an essential fatty acid deficiency that causes a secondary deficiency of "prostaglandin" (very short lived hormones) that control the sodium, chlorides and potassium levels of the sweat!!! Remember the talk by the distinguished anthropologist, Dr. Johnathon Leaky, Sr. who said "the more facts you have, the better the truth you have."

The prevention of CF has been accomplished in pet, farm and laboratory animals by the veterinary profession by assuring adequate levels of selenium and essential fatty acid nutriture to the preconception, pregnant and nursing mother. This is not as easy as it sounds because of malabsorption problems (i.e., celiac diseases and Crohn's Disease) in a percentage of women!!! All things being normal a supplementation of 200 mcg selenium per day and 5 gm of flaxseed oil t.i.d. would be adequate to prevent CF.

Treatment of CF is very basic — treat the infant as early as possible with selenium IM at 10-25 mcg per day. Plant derived colloidal minerals may be used orally thereafter. Provide 5 gm of flaxseed oil orally t.i.d. Most importantly YOU MUST DETERMINE IF THE INFANT IS ALLERGIC TO WHEAT, COW'S MILK OR SOY!!! If you do not correct the malabsorption problem, treatment will only be minimally effective. In the case of older CF patients, IV essential fatty acids and IM selenium provide excellent management leading to a normal life expectancy of 75 years!!! Compare this approach to the heart and lung transplant offered by the "orthodox" pediatricians!!! If the proper treatment is carried out, the "typical CF lung disease" will not develop. The lungs of CF patients are normal at birth and only develop bronchiectasis after chronic essential fatty acid and copper deficiencies have taken their toll. Don't forget the base line nutritional supplementation here!

We went to China in 1988 to study Keshan Disease, a known selenium deficiency disease of Chinese children. We studied 1,700 autopsies and found 595 cases or 35% had pancreatic CF (remember CF is supposed to be "genetic disease of children of middle European extract" — to justify this finding the proponents of the genetic theory will no doubt claim that a very virile English missionary impregnated 125,000 Chinese girls and, unfortunately, he was "carrying the gene for CF."

CYSTITIS (bladder infection): is a common urinary bladder infection in women. Low immune status, improper hygiene habits following bowel movements, pantyhose that are too tight and frequent sexual activity (the reason for the term — "honeymoon disease") are common causes. The symptoms include frequency, urgency and burning on urination. The diagnosis can frequently be made from symptoms alone, however, a urine "dipstick" test will show a positive nitrate test (indicating bacterial infection) and will be positive for a large number of WBCs in the specimen; blood may be present in severe infections (it may also be present during the menstrual period so if the nitrate is negative and no WBCs are present, disregard). In older individuals, cystic calculi (bladder stones) may be considered, especially in males.

Treatment of cystitis consists of acidifying the urine by consuming one to two quarts of cranberry juice per day for the first day then reducing the intake to one quart per day; herbs are very useful and include bearberry (Arctostaphylos uva-ursi), birch (Betula pendula, B. pubescens), juniper (Juniperus communis), lovage (Levisticum officinale), prickly restharrow (Ononis spinosa) and rupture wort (Herniaria glabra).

DANDRUFF: is caused by a change in the surface cells of the scalp which results in a "scaling" or "flaking." This change is caused by one or more nutritional deficiencies. Dandruff may or may not be accompanied by itching.

Treatment of dandruff includes washing the hair in vinegar to remove all of the loose scales. Oral supplementation with flaxseed oil at 5 gm t.i.d., PABA at 100 mg/day, vitamin E at 800-1,200 IU/day, B-6 at 50 mg t.i.d., 300,000 IU vitamin A as beta carotene and zinc at 50 mg t.i.d. and colloidal minerals are recommended.

DEMENTIA (memory loss, as in senile): is a common symptom yet not a true result of aging. Nutritional deficiencies and alcoholism are the common causes of dementia. Symptoms include loss of recent memory, inability to do simple thinking tasks such as math or spelling, losing things, forgetting names, etc. The use of memory enhancing drugs such as hydergine and piracetam will provide excellent prevention of dementia when used to augment good nutrition and supplement program. Don't forget the base line supplement program and colloidal minerals. Check patient for food allergies and hypoglycemia and take appropriate action if either are positive.

Treatment of dementia includes B-1 at 100 mg t.i.d., B-6 at 50 mg t.i.d., B-3 at 450 mg q.i.d. (time release), folic acid at 3-5 mg/day, choline at 500-1,000 mg/day, lecithin at 2,500 mg b.i.d., vitamin E at 800-1,200 IU/day, vitamin C to bowel tolerance, copper at 2-3 mg/day, magnesium at 1,000 mg/day, zinc at 50 mg t.i.d., hydergine at 9 mg/day, vasopressin (Diapid) at 12-16 units/day, centrophenoxine (Lucidril) at 4.4-8.0 gm/day and Piracetam at 2.4-4.8 mg/day, and betaine HCl and pancreatic enzymes at 75-200 mg t.i.d. 15-20 minutes before meals.

DEPRESSION (manic depression): is a common problem in the human population throughout the world — so common that pharmaceutical companies specialize solely in antidepressant drugs. It should be no surprise, however, that very few of the supposedly "expert" psychiatrists ever consider hypoglycemia and food allergies when they do an intake history on a patient who complains of depression. Before you run off and spend $75-$150 per session with a "shrink," do a "pulse test" and a six-hour GTT on yourself (if you're really depressed, you will have to get a family member to help you run these tests to completion. Look for "allergic shiners at the peak of depression. Spontaneous crying, thoughts of suicide and hopelessness are common; depression may be cyclic as in PMS (premenstrual syndrome). Food allergies, hypoglycemia and PMS account for 90% of the diagnosed "depression" today. Avoid caffeine.

Treatment of depression should include dealing with the food allergies (i.e., avoidance, rotation, autoimmune urine/blood therapies) and hypoglycemia (i.e., hypoglycemia diet and chromium/vanadium supplementation at 50-200 mcg t.i.d.; base line supplement program, iron at 45 mg/day, B-6, B-2, B-1 at 50 mg t.i.d., B-12 at 1,000 mcg/day, vitamin C to bowel tolerance, calcium and magnesium at 2,000 mg and 1,000 mg/day, potassium at 250 mg q.i.d., essential fatty acids at 5 gm t.i.d. and dl-phenylalanine, 1-trypto-phane and 1-tyrosine at 2 gm t.i.d. each. Plant derived colloidal minerals with lithium can be useful.

DERMATITIS (atopic, eczema, herpetiformis): is a common form of skin disease but, unfortunately, treated incorrectly by the "orthodox" dermatologists who typically used cortisone or prednisone creams. Ninety-seven percent of these patients have food allergies to wheat gluten, almost equal numbers are sensitive to cow's milk — the scary thing is what you see on the skin is also happening in the lining of your small intestine — the lesions on your skin are a cosmetic problem — the lesions on your intestine area a serious life-threatening absorption problem which, in the end, will deplete your immune system of essential nutrients and result in a variety of serious illnesses (i.e., diabetes, cancer, arthritis, birth defects, etc.).

Atopic dermatitis is characterized by patchy areas of crusty, weeping lesions frequently located on the lips, ears, neck, hands and joints. Atopic dermatitis is very frequently associated with asthma — both together in the same patient is referred to as "atopy" or an "atopic patient."

Eczema is essentially the same lesion as atopic dermatitis but less localized.

Herpetiformis type dermatitis is characterized by clusters of itchy blisters that look like a Herpes eruption.

Hair loss, or alopecia, is a commonly associated problem with any of the above dermatitis and a concurrent essential fatty acid deficiency.

Treatment of all three of the above manifestations of dermatitis should include a gluten free and cow's milk free diet. It is also prudent to do a "pulse test" on frequently consumed foods to determine if they are also affecting you. The supplementation of essential fatty acids are 5 gm q.i.d., PABA at 200 mg q.i.d. and betaine HCl and digestive enzymes at 75-200 mg each t.i.d. before meals should be added on top of the base line supplement program. Have patience, it will take 60-90 days to heal the intestinal lesions to the point where you can absorb nutrients efficiently. Vitamin A at 300,000 IU/day as beta carotene and zinc at 50 mg t.i.d. and colloidal minerals.

DIABETES: is the number one shame of the "orthodox" doctors in the 20th century. Diabetes is easy to prevent, easy to cure and treat so you can avoid all of the terrible side effects (i.e., blindness, hypertension, amputations, early death, etc.). Since 1958, it has been known that supplemental chromium will prevent and treat diabetes as well as hypoglycemia — just ask any health food store owner or N.D.! The facts associated with chromium and diabetes were published in the Federation Proceeding by Walter Mertz (the director of the U.S.D.A. field services). Here is the ultimate case of a whole specialty of medicine being wiped out by universal chromium supplementation but kept secret and away from the public for economic reasons!!! Additionally the University of Vancouver, BC, Canada stated that "Vanadium will replace insulin for adult onset diabetics" !

Chromium/vanadium and the diabetes story should be on the front page of the newspaper in the same bold print as VE DAY instead of any type of artificial heart pump that will save one life for $250,000!!!

The diagnosis of diabetes is very easy and it should be considered in any disease where there is a chronic weight loss or weight gain. Frequent urination and chronic thirst are warning signs that should be explored. A six-hour GTT will show a steep rise of blood glucose at 30-60 minutes to over 275 mg % and may keep rising to over 350 and stay elevated after 4-6 hours. The urine should be tested for sugar with the "dipstick" test every time the blood is tested for sugar. A positive diabetic will always include a positive urine sugar during the six-hour GTT. A morning fasting urine sugar test is useless for the initial diagnosis of diabetes. Blood of the diabetic is also typical in that the lipids and cholesterol are elevated as well as the sugar.

Treatment of diabetes should include chromium and Vanadium at 25 mcg/day in the initial stages to prevent "insulin shock" (sudden dropping of blood sugar because of a relative insulin overdose). Keep checking urine blood sugar before and after meals, as the blood sugar level drops and you can reduce your insulin one or two units per day, go up to 25 mcg b.i.d., then t.i.d.; then go to 50 mcg b.i.d., etc. You will also need to deal with food allergies that cause celiac-type intestinal lesions (i.e., wheat gluten, cow's milk, soya, etc.) and supplement with betaine HCl and digestive enzymes at 75-200 mg t.i.d. before meals. Have patience — the intestinal lesions take 60-90 days to heal.

Treatment of diabetes should also include zinc at 50 mg

t.i.d., B-complex at 50 mg t.i.d. (be sure to include niacin which is part of the GTF "glucose tolerance factor"), essential fatty acids at 5 gm t.i.d., B-12 at 1,000 mcg/day, bioflavonoids including quercetin at 150 mg/day, copper at 2-3 mg/day, lecithin at 2,500 mg t.i.d. and glutathione at 100 mg/day.
High fiber, no processed carbohydrates and avoid meat in the beginning stages of the therapy — the reason is that every time you eat processed carbohydrate (i.e., sugar, honey, alcohol, mashed potatoes, etc.) you will loose 300% more chromium in your urine than when you consume complex carbohydrates! Herbs are useful in treating diabetes and may include licorice (Glycyrrhiza glabra), jaborandi (Pilocarpus jaborandi), yarrow (Achillea Millefolium), Canadian fleabane (Erigeron canadense) and Jerusalem artichoke.

DIAPER RASH: is all too frequent in babies and toddlers, not only because of infrequent changes but also because of food allergies (i.e., wheat, cow's milk, soya, corn, etc.). Do a pulse test on babies as you introduce them to new foods (be sure to test the old ones, too), use avoidance or rotation diet systems, B-6 at 5-25 mg t.i.d., zinc at 5-15 mg b.i.d. and vitamin E oil and/or aloe vera topically. Plant derived colloidal minerals are fantastic for diabetics!

DIARRHEA (dysentery): can be caused by simply eating too much of a good thing (i.e., fruit, juices, etc.), food allergies (i.e., celiac disease, strawberries, fish, etc.), soap ingestion from improperly rinsed dishes or can indicate a more serious problem such as parasites, food poisoning or even cancer. Knowledge of your own body and how it reacts is important here as you will have to sort things out — did you go to an apple farm yesterday and eat a peck of apples? Have you had diarrhea since your trip to Mexico? What medications are you on? Have you been losing weight and have diarrhea off and on for six months? If the latter, you may consider "irritable bowel syndrome" or the more serious cancer — at any rate you should consider a "lower GI" or a colonoscopic exam. Treatment for simple diarrhea can include commercial products such as Pepto Bismol or Kaopectate, charcoal capsules, fiber, and herbs including American blackberry (Rubus villosus), barley (Hordeum distichon), clove root (Geumur-banum), whortleberry (Vaccinium myrtillus), black currant (Ribes nigrum), hounds tongue (Cynoglossum officinale), Lady's mantle (Alchemilla vulgaris) and tormentil blood root (Potentilla erecta).

DIETING (weight loss): is a common practice in the western world because "thin is in." There are some basic habits that will help the weight loss effort and help keep the weight off:

1) First, avoid caffeine as it causes a drop in blood sugar 30-90 minutes after consumption and thus creates "hunger pangs."

2) Drink eight (8) glasses of water each day as many trips to the ice box are caused by thirst rather than hunger and a restricted diet doesn't decrease your need for water but does reduce your water intake from food.

3) Diagnose any health problems you may have such as addictive food allergies (pulse test), hypoglycemia (six-hour GTT) or hypothyroidism (basal body temperature) that might contribute to a weight problem.

4) Don't skip meals — eat a breakfast like a Queen (or King), lunch like a princess (or prince) and dinner like a pauper. Stay on a meal schedule; if you are going out to eat, don't skip a meal but rather have one of those high fiber/low cal drinks or food bars to assure a limited calo-

rie intake — then enjoy your dinner date!!! Remember, in the long run it's the basic habits that will help you lose weight and keep it off.
5) Exercise, if done in moderation and on a schedule, will help you loose weight and not make you overly hungry for a snack — eat a piece of fruit or have some nuts after exercise; don't wait three hours until your next meal to eat or drink. The plant derived colloidal minerals are excellent after event refreshers.
6) Before meal fibers (i.e., oat bran diet tabs) taken with eight ounces of water 30 minutes before meals will help curb appetite.
7) Don't forget the base line supplements — remember restricted diets restrict nutrients and result in pica and cribbing. Plant derived colloidal minerals are fantastic here!
8) Essential fatty acids in the form of flaxseed oil at 5 gm t.i.d. will help regulate and normalize fat metabolism.
9) Thyroid will help if your basal body temperature is low (below 97.6°F). Too much will cause increase in basal pulse rate and make you speedy and unable to sleep — start out with 1/2 gr. and cut back or add to as needed.
10) If you do all of the above, you will be slim, slim, slim!!!

DIURETIC: broom-corn (Sorghum vulgare)

DIURETIC & LAXATIVE: asparagus (Asparagus officinalis)

DIURETIC & CATHARTIC: broom (Cystisus scoparius)

DIVERTICULITIS: is an inflammation of the small pea sized sacs in the outerwall of the colon. This inflammation is the result of a low fiber diet over a long period of time which allows tiny concretions to build up to a size that does not allow them to exit into the colon. These concretions irritate the colon wall to the point of causing painful spasm. Prevention includes high fiber diet (i.e., oat bran, 4-6 cups of vegetables per day, etc.). Certain foods, including corn, peanuts and raw carrots can result in severe spasms. Rarely is blood detected in the stool with uncomplicated diverticulitis. Diverticulitis is easily diagnosed with a lower GI series.

Treatment of diverticulitis includes colonics two to three times per week, high fiber diet, eight glasses of water per day and regular exercise.

DOUCHE: is a useful feminine hygiene practice, especially if one has a history of discharges or infection. Retention douches are particularly effective — this is accomplished best in a bathtub with the feet up on the sides to aid in retaining the fluid for 10-15 minutes. Use 4-8 oz. of diluted vinegar (4 oz/pint of warm distilled water, 1 1/2% hydrogen peroxide (4-8 oz.), bayberry myrtle (Myrica cerifera) (one oz. powdered bark to one pint water — warm to body temperature), and numerous commercial products. Plain unsweetened yogurt or Superdolph capsules emptied into warm water (10-20 per 4 oz.) maybe used to replant Lactobacillus acidophilus to normalize flora after vaginitis and/or antibiotic therapy.

DROPSY (water belly, abdominal edema): is a common occurrence in chronic kidney, liver or heart disease and cancer. Low protein diets will also result in "dropsy." "Dropsy" is fluid accumulating in the belly cavity because the protein content of the blood is so low that fluid can't be held in the blood vessels (an osmotic gradient); poor circulation because of liver or heart disease is also a common cause.

Treatment of dropsy should include an improvement of the protein level of the blood, IV amino acids and the basic health of the liver, kidneys and heart and diuresis. Herbs are particularly useful and may include foxglove (Digitalis purpurea) - BE CAREFUL HERE; THIS PLANT IS POTENTIALLY DANGEROUS, lily-of-the-valley (Convallaria magalis), English hawthorne (Crataegus oxycanthus), Canadian fleabane (Erigeron canadense), kidney bean (Phaseolus vulgaris), Scotch broom (Cystisus scoparius), parsley (Petroselinum crispum), prickly restharrow (Ononis Spinosa) and nettle (Urtica urens).

DRY SKIN: is a common malady in the western world; it, in itself, is a cosmetic problem; however, it is a signal of a potentially more serious problem — essential fatty acid deficiency that can result in cardiovascular disease (i.e., stroke, heart attack, etc.). Superficial creams will temporarily deal with the superficial problem but the more ominous results of the bodies deficiency of essential fatty acids can be sudden and deadly!!! DSM/EFA or "dry skin means essential fatty acids"!!! If you are supplementing with more than 50,000-100,000 units of vitamin A, dry skin may signal the early stages of vitamin A overdose.

Treatment of dry skin includes flaxseed oil orally at 5 gm t.i.d., B-6 at 50 mg t.i.d., zinc at 50 mg t.i.d., vitamin E at 800-1,200 IU/day and if you are not supplementing vitamin A in excess, use vitamin A at 300,000 units/day as beta carotene.

DUMPING SYNDROME: is the sudden "dumping" of stomach contents into the small intestine all at once, thus overloading the natural intestinal buffer system. The resulting acid conditions in the intestine prevents proper functioning of pancreatic enzymes which require an alkaline environment. Dumping syndrome is a common side effect of stomach surgery. Anemia and osteoporosis are common secondary diseases of the dumping syndrome.

Treatment of the dumping syndrome should include any of the classic "bitters" (i.e., gentian, Gentiana lutea), folic acid at 3-5 mg/day, pectin at 1/2 oz. in water before meals, high animal protein diets, and you should lay down for a half hour after meals. Don't forget the base line supplements here!!!

DYSENTERY (diarrhea): is characterized by a watery projectile diarrhea that creates cramping, urgency and exhaustion from loss of electrolytes. Causes of dysentery range widely from "too rich" a diet (usually too much party — such as wine, lobster, creamy desserts, etc.), improperly stored food that results in bacterial overgrowth, food poisoning, food allergies (i.e., celiac disease), etc. Prevention of dysentery requires attention to details of food storage, hygiene, self-discipline, and preparation.

If you have a busy schedule that can't be altered, you will have to resort to commercial products such as Pepto-Bismol or Kaopectate (fortunately, they have tablets that you can quietly carry with you on your errands). Weak black tea, rice water, lime water, chicken broth or bouillon to replace electrolytes (another good source are the athletic "thirst quenchers." Herbs such as Irish moss (Chondrus crispus) and common ivy (Hedera helix) are of great benefit in quieting the run away colon!!!

DYSLEXIA (learning disorder, hyperactivity): is a complex syndrome rather than a specific disease. To be sure, there are some dyslexic children who have true organic or biochemical brain injury who will require intense "special" education and training programs; however, it is a sad testimony to American "orthodox" medicine that as many as 80% of these "dyslexic" kids are really suffering from food allergies and/or sugar sensitivity (where sugar acts as a drug and produces a "pharmacological effect" just like "speed"). These food sensitivities create learning disabilities that "mimic" organic disease and too many salvageable kids are put on drugs (i.e., Ritalin), shunted off into "special" education programs or worse yet, given up on as "lost" by frightened, frustrated families. Food allergies and sensitivities should be seriously investigated and dealt with (i.e., pulse test, elimination diets and diet diaries) if these children are to have a fair shot at a normal life.

I speak with a great deal of experience with this problem as my youngest son was deemed to be a "learning disabled" child (zero brain waves would be a better description — at age six he couldn't print his first name or count to ten). To make a long story short, he was cured in two weeks by eliminating sugar, milk, wheat and corn from his diet. His teachers were convinced that I had exchanged him with his "normal" twin — they couldn't believe such a turn around with just a dietary program!!! To condemn a "dyslexia" child without investigating food allergies and sensitivities is equal to finding an innocent man "guilty" of murder and sentenced to life in prison — what a waste and what a tragedy!!!

Treatment and prevention are closely intertwined. Digestive enzymes and betaine HCl are essential to prevent progression of the problem as well as aid in onset of symptoms. The "Feingold Diet" is a good place to start, however, it, in itself, is not a "shield" to be totally relied upon. There are many foods and food additives not excluded by the Feingold program that will set off some kids like sky rockets (we had one dyslexic child patient that did everything the Feingold Diet required except eliminate honey — we found him on top of a 40 foot dome!). Rotation diets, allergy elimination diets and autoimmune urine therapy should be aggressively pursued — the rewards are beyond your wildest expectations.

DYSMENORRHEA (menstrual pain): is a common event in western women, so common that it is frequently considered part of PMS. Sometimes the discomfort of dysmenorrhea is intense enough to be debilitating. There are a number of excellent commercial products that will dampen the pain but not deal with the basic problem — an abnormal prostaglandin metabolism.

Treatment includes B-3 and B-6 at 50-100 mg t.i.d., calcium and magnesium at 2,000 and 1,000 mg/day, vitamin E at 800-1,200 IU/day, essential fatty acids at 5 gm t.i.d. Don't forget the base line nutritional supplements and avoid caffeine. Herbs such as blue cohosh (Caulophyllum thalictroides) and black cohosh (Cimicifuga racemosa) are the ideal natural approach to pain of dysmenorrhea.

DYSPEPSIA (poor digestion, indigestion): is characterized by "belching, bloating, burping" and "acid stomach." Dyspepsia is probably the most common "disease" in the western world and is certainly the most costly from the amount of money spent on "relief." Even more costly is the secondary results of chronic dyspepsia (i.e., food allergies, osteoporosis, anemia, debilitated immune system, degenerative disease!!!). Prevention includes reduced stress levels, exercise, healthful diet habits and reasonable food volumes. An unforgiving event as we age is a decrease in stomach acid production, the main cause of dyspepsia in seniors, prevention in this case includes the regular use of digestive aids.

Treatment of dyspepsia includes supplementation of 75-200 mg betaine HCl and pancreatic enzymes t.i.d. 15-30 minutes before each meal (the "acid" is not acid enough and is burped up with bacterially generated gas), "antacids" are a good "temporary fix" in an emergency (regular use will eventually damage you), herbal preventions and remedies include papaya (Carica papaya), common barberry (Berberis vulgaris) and bitters such as gentian (Gentiana lutea). In some cases, a glass of wine or several oz. of vinegar before meals will be helpful.

EARACHE (ear infections): tonsillitis, sinusitis and bronchitis are related in cause, prevention and cure. Allergies to cow's milk is the most frequent common denominator, so well does it mimic strep throat (including pain and fever) that most "orthodox" doctors will prescribe penicillin syrup for affected children over the phone!!! The "orthodox" EENT will want to surgically place "tubes" in the ears of infants and toddlers to treat "chronic earaches." Simple avoidance of cow's milk and cow's milk products will prevent chronic "earaches" and tonsillitis.

Treatment of milk allergy "earaches" and tonsillitis includes avoidance of milk and milk products, avoidance of sugar, treat fever and discomfort with demulcents and antipyretics (i.e., willow, Salix alba), hydrogen peroxide eardrops and/or mullein oil drops (Verbascum thapsus). Treat as with any allergy including autoimmune urine therapy. True strep throat requires the use of penicillin.

ECCHYMOSIS (easy bruising): is very common, especially in women and children on low fiber, low fruit and

low vegetable diets (i.e., fast foods, lots of coffee, tea and soft drinks).
Treatment includes alfalfa tablets at 4-6 b.i.d., vitamin C to bowel tolerance, vitamin K at 15 mg/day, vitamin E at 800-1,200 IU/day and 4-6 cups of green vegetables each day.

ECZEMA (atopic dermatitis, psoriasis): is a dry patchy scale on localized skin areas (i.e., ears, nose, joints, breasts, etc.). Eczema is usually the result of food allergies, especially cow's milk, wheat and soy. Do pulse tests and elimination diets to determine the culprits. This is not only a cosmetic problem as the same damage is occurring in the intestinal lining which can lead to malabsorption, lowered immune status and chronic degenerative diseases.
Treatment includes avoidance of offending foods, autoimmune urine therapy, betaine HCl and pancreatic enzymes at 75-200 mg t.i.d. before meals each day, folic acid at 3-5 mg/day, essential fatty acids at 5 mg t.i.d., vitamin A at 300,000 IU/day as beta carotene, zinc at 50 mg t.i.d., vitamin C at bowel tolerance and vitamin E at 800-1200 IU/day; topical herbs include aloe vera (Aloe spp.), wild strawberry (Fragaria vesca), araroba (andira araroba) and Labrador tea (Ledum latifolium), comfrey (Symphytum officinale), English walnut (Juglans regia), European snakeroot (Aristolochia clematitis), flaxseed or linseed oil (Linum usitatisimum), German chamomile (Matricaria chamomilla), great burdock (Arctium lappa), high mallow (Malvia sylvestris), hounds tongue (Cynoglossum officinale), marigold (Calendula officinalis), oak (Quercus robur) and pansy (Viola tricolor); Dermese orally, IM or topically gives great results.

EJACULATION (premature): is a common problem in

today's busy world. Premature ejaculation is usually equated as "poor performance" on the part of the male, however, can easily be prevented and cured if both the "guy" and "doll" understand the basic cause. Again "orthodox" sexologist would have you believe that there is a "mental block" or some "deep seated guilt trip" that you have to deal with — anything to keep you coming again (pardon the pun). The true basics of premature ejaculation (it happens to all men given the classic circumstances) include a mental state of high expectation, infrequency of sex and too much friction. The "orthodox" approach to therapy is to "think of draining your car's oil" so you're not thinking of sex (how absurd can you get) how can you participate in the sex act and not be aware of sex — who would want to?

Treatment and prevention of premature ejaculation are interrelated. The most important part of the treatment is to be very open about you and your "doll's" body (have you ever wondered why hippie gurus were so good at sex?). Spend a lot of time together naked, take showers together, read in bed together naked on top of the covers, have sex in any room (obviously you have to make sure the kids are somewhere else), give each other massages (both naked) until the sight of each other's naked body is no big deal.

Step number two is to have frequent sex; this definitely requires effort by both the "guy" and the "doll." Frequent sex means two to three times per night three to four nights per week. This is easier than it sounds when both are cooperating. The "doll" can't expect the "guy" to give a marathon performance once each week when she's in a high demand state but has been fending the "guy" off all week because she is into shopping with the girls or taking the kids to ballet, aerobics, movies and grandma's. For the "guy's" part, he can't expect the "doll" to be receptive regularly if he isn't "romantic" (i.e., kindness, flowers, dancing, gifts, compliments, wine, perfume, shower, shave, after-shave — you know, just like when you were courting) — the "wham, bam, thank you, ma'am" just isn't attractive to the "dolls."

The third aspect of preventing and curing premature ejaculation is lubrication. The "guy" must make sure that the "doll" is properly lubricated. This can be accomplished in many ways, including the "doll's" natural lubrication that results from emotional excitement and sexual stimulation. If the "doll" is a slow responder, the "guy" can liberally cover his penis with a water soluble gel (i.e., K-Y Jelly) as well as apply some to the vaginal opening. Slowly insert the penis into the vagina and just "let it soak." After awhile, the "doll" relaxes and the "guy" can move around a little without premature ejaculation. This is one process that there are no short cuts for (who would want any??!!). Herbs, ginseng (Panax spp.) and herb combinations (Zumba) are excellent tonifying agents for increasing the "guy's" potency.

ELECTRIC SHOCK: can be fatal, even with the 110 electric outlets in the home. Toddlers sticking bobby pins or keys into the outlet can have a fatal shock, radios or appliances falling into the bathtub can be fatal to adults as can electrical repairs without turning off the breakers. Electricity kills by disrupting the electrical signals of the heart's regulating mechanism which causes the heart to "fibrillate" (quiver rather than beat normally) and the breathing muscles to become paralyzed.

Treatment of electric shock includes shutting off the source of electricity or breaking the electrical contact with the patient and reestablishing the basic functions of life with CPR (cardio pulmonary resuscitation) and oxygen. HAVE SOMEONE CALL 911 FOR EMERGENCY HELP!

EMESIS (vomiting): is a distressing event that may indicate overeating, cancer, excessive alcohol consumption, poisoning, food poisoning, food allergies, infection (i.e., flu, EBV, Candida, etc.). In infants, vomiting with lethargy (unresponsive) and fever can be an ominous signal indicating meningitis. You may wish to cause vomiting when a child (or adult, for that matter) consumes a noncorrosive poison (i.e., rat poisons, toxic plants, household chemicals, etc.). "Coffee grounds" vomiting indicates large amounts of blood from a bleeding ulcer and/or stomach cancer and is a critical sign as death from uncontrolled bleeding can occur — seek emergency help here. Early pregnancy often times will be heralded by nausea and vomiting ("morning sickness").
Treatment of vomiting can be simply to not eat for several hours, suck ice, drink small amounts of peppermint tea, drink small amounts of chicken or beef bouillon. Drinking small volumes of athletic fluid/electrolyte replacers is of value. If stomach irritation is severe don't be bashful about taking Pepto Bismol or Kaopectate — preferably the liquid to coat the stomach.
To cause vomiting in case of noncorrosive poisoning including drug ingestion, you can use the ipecac syrup from your home "pharmacy" at 1 tbsp. for children and 2 tbsp. for adults; have the patient take in a large amount of water (one quart for an adult and as much as one pint for a child); repeat the dose in 15 minutes if necessary.

ENURESIS (bedwetting): in children is another one of those outrageous syndromes botched by the "orthodox" pediatrician or, worse yet, the psychiatrist!! The "orthodox" view of enuresis is that it is "genetic," associated with "passive-aggressive" behavior, "dependency," "sleepwalking," "anti-social behavior," and "speech disorders."

Enuresis is, in fact, the result of food allergies (i.e., sugar, milk, etc.) and/or severe reactive hypoglycemia; calcium/ magnesium deficiencies complicate the food allergies and hypoglycemia. All the behavioral symptoms associated with enuresis are pretty typical of "hyperactivity" which again is caused by the food allergies and/ or the hypoglycemia, combined with unnatural interest in fire and cruel behavior. Bedwetting is a serious sign of future violent behavior. Employ the pulse test and a six-hour GTT to get a complete picture of the cause.

Treatment of enuresis includes eliminating the offending foods for food allergies, eliminating sugar (including sweet juices, i.e., grape and apple) from bedtime treats, digestive aids (i.e., betaine HCl and pancreatic enzymes) at 75-200 mg t.i.d. 15-20 minutes before meals, calcium and magnesium at 2,000 mg and 1,000 mg; don't forget the base line supplement program and colloidal minerals.

EPILEPSY (fits, convulsions): is classically categorized by severity: 1) "petite mal," or small seizure, is often times a blank stare or dizziness that comes over the patient for but a brief moment; 2) "grand mal," or large seizures, are spectacular convulsive attacks where the patient becomes stiff, falls over and begins to gnash his teeth and "flop" or "jerk" around the floor. The "grand mal" seizure can be fatal if the patient vomits and inhales the vomitus or hits his head; tongue biting commonly occurs.

Treatment of epilepsy by the "orthodox" doctor will include the use of phenytoin at 5-10 mg/kg in children and 300-500 mg in adults, phenobarbital at 5-10 mg/kg in children and 2-5 mg/kg in adults, and premidone at 10-20 mg/kg in children and 0.75-1.5 gm in adults (may need to increase slowly). These allopathic drugs will stop symptomatic convulsions, however, they do have dramatic and potentially dangerous side effects (i.e., uncontrolled eye movements, weakness and stumbling, arthritis and osteoporosis, skin rashes and/or dermatitis, anemia, learning disabilities and hyperactivity. Vitamin B-6 alone will frequently "cure" epilepsy at 50-100 mg t.i.d. (long term administration can cause some numbness and tingling in the face or hands), calcium magnesium at 2,000 and 1,000 mg/day, folic acid at 15-25 mg/day and B-12 at 1,000 mcg/day IM can also be curative, manganese at 50 mg/day, zinc at 50 mg t.i.d., essential fatty acids at 5 gm t.i.d., choline at 4 gm/day, taurine at 500 mg t.i.d. and dimethyl glycine at 100 mg b.i.d.

EXOPHTHALMOS (bug eyes): is a prominent protrusion of the eyes from any of several causes including hyperthyroidism, tumor (especially if only one eye is affected) or glaucoma.
Treatment is specifically related to the cause. Blood test for thyroid function, glaucoma exam and consideration of brain tumor (orbital or eye) is indicated.

EYE REDNESS (sties, pink eye): can be caused by dust, pollen allergies, bright sunshine, overwork, irritants (i.e., cigarette smoke), staying up late, infection, foreign body, etc.).
Treatment of the eyes should be taken seriously. Infection can be treated with ophthalmic ointments with either boric acid or neomycin from your home "pharmacy," commercial eye drops such as Visine work very well for simple irritation, pulling the upper eyelid outward and over the lower lid will cause enough tear flow to wash out small foreign bodies such as eyelashes and dust, herbs can be used for eye washes including eyebright

(Euphrasia rostkoviana), fennel (Foeniculum vulgare), German chamomile (Matricaria chamomilla), oak (Quercus robur), pasque flower (Pulsatilla vulgaris) and cornflower (Centaurea cyanus).

FAILURE TO THRIVE: is a term used to describe an infant that falls below expected growth rates. Celiac disease and/or other food allergies and cystic fibrosis should be considered as the most common cause. Plant derived colloidal minerals are of great value here as most of these children are severely depleted in trace minerals and rare earths.

FARTING (bowel gas): is usually caused by digested but poorly absorbed food reaching the colon and being fermented by bowel organisms. Some foods such as beans, garlic and onions are legendary in the production of bowel gas. Food allergies can cause celiac disease type changes in the small intestine which results in malabsorption.

Treatment for pathological amounts of unpleasant bowel gas includes the avoidance of offending foods, betaine HCl and pancreatic enzymes at 75-200 mg t.i.d. 15-20 minutes before meals and autoimmune urine therapy where food allergies have caused celiac disease type changes in the small intestine.

FATIGUE (chronic fatigue syndrome, Candidiasis, Epstein-Barr Virus, cytomegalovirus, human herpes 6 virus, human B lymphotrophic virus, food allergies, hypoglycemia, diabetes, anemia, malnutrition): is the disease of the 80s. SEE SPECIFIC DISEASE DESCRIPTION.

Treatment should be specific as described in appropriate section; in addition, herbs may be of value including

American ginseng (Panax quinquefolius), lavender (Lavandula augustifolia), rosemary (Rosmarinus officinalis), sweet flag (Acorus calamus) and pasque flower (Anemone pulsatilla).

FERTILITY (problems): that are not related to physical blockage of egg or sperm transport systems are usually the result of some form of malnutrition, either overt (i.e., diet fads) or secondary to food allergies and/or malabsorption. One also must be sure that the woman is cycling and ovulating properly (i.e., slim women with less than 20% body fat do not ovulate regularly). Infertility usually means that the condition can be reversed whereas sterility usually means permanent nonreversible conditions. Do hair analysis and pulse test.
Treatment of this form of infertility includes the base line nutritional supplement, pay special attention to selenium deficiency in male infertility, betaine HCl and pancreatic enzymes at 75-200 mg t.i.d. before meals, correction of quality protein intake to a minimum of 80 gm/day (the RDA is only 40 gm/day) and essential fatty acids at 5 gm t.i.d.

FEVER: or elevated temperature (normal is 98.6°F) is part of the bodies defense mechanism; many enzymes, antibodies and cell (WBCs) responses are more efficient in slightly elevated temperatures. Elevated temperature during the day is not bad per se but should be reduced at night to allow comfortable sleep. Infants with high fevers of 104°F or above may have convulsions which must be reduced quickly by immersion in tepid water.
Treatment of fever can include a number of commercial products including aspirin, Tylenol, Nuprin, etc., ice packs on the forehead, running cool water over the wrists, cool baths and herbs to include feverfew (Chrysanthe-

mum parthenium), meadow-sweet (Filipendula ulmaria), sea buckthorn (Hippophae rhamnoides), European holly (Ilex aquifolium), white willow (Salix alba), mugwort (Artemisia vulgaris) and cinchona bark (Cinchona succirubra). Obviously, all of the above are symptomatic treatments; the basic disease process (i.e., cold, flu, pneumonia, cancer, etc.) must also be dealt with forthrightly.

FIBROCYSTIC BREAST DISEASE: is cosmetically unpleasant and often painful during peak estrogen production. Cyst may vary in size from pea size to grapes and occasionally larger. Prevention and treatment are the same course of action.

Treatment of fibrocystic breast disease includes avoiding methyl xanthines (i.e., caffeine, coffee, black tea, ice tea, carbonated soft drinks with caffeine, chocolate, sugar, etc.), vitamin E at 800-1,200 IU/day, vitamin A at 300,000 IU/day as beta carotene, essential fatty acids at 5 gm t.i.d., iodine at 200 mcg/day, selenium at 500 mcg/day.

FIBROMYALGIA (stiff lamb disease, adult onset muscular dystrophy): is a disease that was eliminated from lambs in 1957. It is a multiple deficiency disease caused by a high intake of fried foods and vegetable oils (margarine, cooking oils and salad dressing) and deficiencies of selenium, vitamin E and sulfur amino acids (methionine, mysteine, cystene).

Treatment includes eliminating all vegetable oils and fried foods and supplementation with selenium 500 mcg, vitamin E 1200 i,u, and an amino acid program that includes methionine, cysteine and cystine.

FINGERNAILS (white spots, ridges, brittle): are good barometers of absorption and nutritional status. Bluish fingernails indicate chronic lung conditions (i.e., not enough oxygen), white spots indicate zinc deficiency, ridges can indicate iron and/or calcium deficiency and brittle nails indicates sulfur amino acid deficiencies. Don't forget the base line nutritional supplements.

Treatment of fingernail problems should include gelatin (diabetic Jello, or Knox gelatin) — this is especially important for those who have been vegetarians for any length of time, essential fatty acids at 5 gm t.i.d. and betaine HCl and pancreatic enzymes at 75-200 mg t.i.d. before meals.

FITS (see epilepsy): can be caused by a variety of problems including epilepsy, high fever in children and certain poisons. See epilepsy. You may wish to call your local poison center "hotline" for poisoning — keep the telephone number taped on your telephone, especially if you have small children. In addition to the medications indicated for epilepsy, you may consider mullein tea (Verbascum thapsus).

FLATULENCE (bowel gas, colic, farting): is a signal that unabsorbed foods, especially proteins, are reaching the colon where they are fermented by colon organisms. Do the pulse test to see if any allergies are present that might cause celiac changes in the small intestine.

Treatment of flatulence includes digestive enzymes at 75-200 mg t.i.d. 15-20 minutes before meals, avoidance and/or rotation of offending food allergens, autoimmune urine therapy and herbs including angelica (Angelica archangelica), anise (Pimpinella anisum), caraway (Carum carvi), dill (Anethum graveolens), fennel (Foeniculum vulgare) and pepper (Piper nigrum).

FLU (influenza, grip): is a potentially fatal viral disease;

infants and elder citizens are susceptible to the most serious effects if they are poorly nourished, immune comprised or have a serious respiratory ailment (i.e., emphysema, asthma, pneumonia, CF, etc.). Flu is characterized by prostration, fever, diarrhea, bronchitis, coughing, headache, pneumonia, muscle aches, joint aches and chills (feel cold and shaky but sweating). Flu typically occurs as a winter epidemic; vaccination is very questionable for several reasons: 1) there are numerous strains and serotypes of flu virus (perhaps thousands!) so a vaccine for one strain or serotype is a "crap shoot" at best — usually you will come up "snake eyes" and get vaccinated for the wrong strain; 2) carte blanche vaccination has been identified as the probable vehicle for a variety of human epidemics including the first wave of AIDS!; 3) damage to the brain and nervous system.

Treatment for the flu includes antiviral agents such as Ribavirin at 1-2 tablets q.i.d. and/or Isoprinosin at 1 capsule b.i.d.; Fluviatol is another good choice at 2 tablets q.i.d. (pregnant women should avoid these products because they potentially can cause birth defects), you will also want to include some protection against secondary bacterial pneumonia (i.e., Staphylococcus or Pneumococcus) such as echinacea (Echinacea angustifolia) or golden seal (Hydrastis canadensis); individuals with low immune status or severe respiratory disease may choose to take antibiotics rather than a vaccine. Fluids (i.e., juices, chicken/rice soup, vegetable soup, etc.) are essential to prevent dehydration and replace electrolytes lost through diarrhea or vomiting. Vitamin C to bowel tolerance (if you already have diarrhea, take 1,000 mg time release tablets hourly during your waking day), vitamin A at 300,000 IU/day as beta carotene, bioflavonoids at 150-300 mg/day, zinc at 50 mg t.i.d., ACE (adrenal cortical extract sublingual or IV), herbs including wormwood

(Artemisia absinthium), cinchona bark (Cinchona succirubra), eucalyptus (Eucalyptus globulus), hemp acrimony (Eupatorium cannabinum) meadowsweet (Filipendula ulmaria), sea buckthorn (Hippophae rhamnoides), European holly (Ilex aquifolium), dog rose (Rosa canina), white willow (Salix alba), European elder (Sambucus nigra), broad-leafed lime (Tilia platyphllos) and bearded usnea (Usnea barbata).

FOOD ALLERGIES (sensitivities): are a concern for everyone. The reason is that the celiac disease type changes they cause in your intestines will prevent the absorption of essential nutrients that are required to keep your immune system, as well as your various organs, in tip top working order. Many of the maladies caused by food allergies are not a direct cause but rather an indirect cause by cutting off the flow of essential raw materials necessary for your body to repair itself. A list of symptoms of food allergies would perhaps fill ten pages of this book - suffice it to be said that if you have any chronic disease (i.e., cancer, diabetes, arthritis, heart disease, etc.) and/or emotional problems (i.e., hypoglycemia, depression, neurosis, schizophrenia, hyperactivity, paranoia, etc.) you have food allergies! Allergic "shiners" and "geographic" tongue are red flags. Food allergies are caused by incompletely digested proteins (polypeptides) getting into your blood stream; this happens to the fetus through the placenta (i.e., cystic fibrosis, celiac disease, etc.), to the nursing baby through the breast milk and to the rest of us when our digestive system is not working perfectly (i.e., stress, aging, etc.).

The diagnosis and identification of specific food allergens takes quite a bit of work on your part to identify but it is worth the effort as it will add 10-20 years to your life and make an enormous improvement in your quality of life. The easiest way to identify food allergies in yourself is the Coca Pulse Test. To perform this test, you learn your base pulse rate then eat a single food (i.e., milk only, wheat only, etc.) and check your pulse 15, 30 and 60 minutes after you eat the single food item; an elevation in pulse rate of more than ten beats is an indicator that you are allergic to that food. You must be serious and aggressive at this project because it takes time and effort — after you get cancer, it is a little late to realize that you spent more time working on your lawns health than you did on your own!!! A second method of allergy diagnosis can be used in conjunction with the pulse test is the diet diary; this is especially useful when emotional symptoms and headache are associated with food allergies. First, you eat a single food (do with pulse test) noting the time on a pad of paper, then record emotional symptoms and/or headache with the time; the symptom will appear within minutes to a few hours of ingesting the offending food (this includes hyperactivity and dyslexia). Do a six-hour GTT as almost everyone with food allergies has hypoglycemia because the celiac changes in the intestine prevent the efficient absorption of chromium.

Treatment of food allergies includes religious use of the base line nutritional supplements (be sure to use hypoallergenic supplements — no corn, wheat, soy, egg or milk), avoid vaccinations that have egg, blood or beef origins; vitamin C to bowel tolerance levels, vitamin A at 300,000 IU/day as beta carotene, bioflavonoids at 150-300 mg/day, zinc at 50 mg t.i.d., essential fatty acids at 5 gm t.i.d., selenium at 200 mcg t.i.d., chromium at 50-200 mcg t.i.d., betaine HCl and pancreatic enzymes at 75-500 mg t.i.d. 15-20 minutes before meals, ACE sublingual or IV, autoimmune urine therapy, five day rotation diets, avoidance of offending foods and patience!!! It takes up to 90 days to repair the intestinal injury (the good news is that repair will take place even if you're 100 years old!!!). IV hydrogen peroxide speeds up the healing process.

FRACTURES (broken bones): can result from malnutrition (i.e., calcium/magnesium deficiency, improper calcium/phosphorus ratio; osteoporosis) severe trauma (i.e., a blow during a fight, auto accident, fall, etc.); however, good mineral status in your bones will prevent most types of "spontaneous" fractures and fractures from simple falls. Diagnosis of a fracture can be made by seeing a digit or limb at an abnormal angle, noticing severe pain at a specific place on the bone, use a vibrating tuning fork to touch the suspected fracture site; the vibrations will be painful if there is a fracture present. X-rays in an emergency room may be warranted to differentiate between a fracture and a sprain or strain. The use of the base line nutritional supplements including calcium and magnesium at 2,000 mg and 1,000 mg per day, plant derived colloidal minerals and digestive aids (i.e., betaine HCl and pancreatic enzymes at 75-200 mg t.i.d. before meals) is an almost sure guarantee against nontrauma fractures especially in post-menopause women. The use of comfrey (Symphytum officinale) orally and over the injury site will speed healing of fractures as well as reduce pain and swelling.

FRECKLES (liver spots): are caused by melanin pigment in response to sunlight in fair skinned people; "liver spots" in middle aged and older people are sometimes difficult to distinguish from freckles; liver spots are caused by "ceroid" pigment build up in the skin from peroxidation of fats in your body (i.e., free radical damage) and are a more ominous sign than freckles. Freckles may be prevented or reduced by the religious use of sun screens by fair skinned people.

Treatment of freckles and "liver spots" includes the use of vitamin E at 800-1,200 IU/day, selenium at 200-500 mcg t.i.d., vitamin C to bowel tolerance, vitamin A at 300,000 IU/day as beta carotene, essential fatty acids at 5 gm t.i.d. and the herb, English mandrake (Tamus communis) topically on the spots b.i.d.

GALLBLADDER DISEASE (gall stones): is generally caused by liver problems, especially with fat and cholesterol metabolism. Gallbladder "attacks" are caused by a cramping of the muscles in the gallbladder after a fatty meal or a temporary blockage of the bile duct by a gallstone. Gallstones are composed of cholesterol and fat when they first form and become calcified after the passage of time. Prevention of gallbladder problems includes the use of glycyrrhizin (an extract of the licorice plant, Glycyrrhyza glabra), the base line nutritional supplement including 5 gm of essential fatty acids t.i.d. Eggs are known to precipitate 93% of all gallbladder attacks, followed closely by onions and pork.

Treatment of gallbladder disease and gallstones includes the use of high fiber diets (i.e., make sure you are having 2-3 bowel movements per day), lecithin at 2,500 mg t.i.d., essential fatty acids at 5 gm t.i.d., vitamin E at 800-1,200 IU per day, vitamin C to bowel tolerance, selenium at 200 mcg t.i.d., and taurine at 500 mg t.i.d. Virgin olive oil in eight oz. of grapefruit or lemon juice will help to flush liver; herbs include acrimony (Agrimonia eupatoria), blessed thistle (Cnicus benedictus), vumitory (Fumaria officinalis), horehound (Marrubium vulgare), licorice (Glycyrrhiza glabra), peppermint (Mentha piperita), wormwood (Artemisia absinthium), artichoke (Cynara scolymus), sweet coltsfoot (Petasites hybridus), celandine (Chelidonium majus), chicory (Cichorium intybus), and dandelion (Taraxacum officinale).

GEOGRAPHIC TONGUE (benign migratory glossitis): like allergic "shiners" is a red flag that you are not absorbing B-3, B-2, B-6, B-5, B-12, folic acid or zinc (the cause is usually malabsorption from celiac disease-like changes in the small intestine). Geographic tongue is recognized by irregular denuded areas on the top surface and sides of the tongue. Do a series of pulse tests to determine what foods you may be allergic to. Geographic tongue is not painful and taste may or may not be affected. Treatment of geographic tongue includes avoidance of any offending food allergens, autoimmune urine therapy, zinc at 50 mg t.i.d., betaine HCl and pancreatic enzymes at 75-200 mg t.i.d. before meals, B-complex IM in the early stages of therapy, be sure to get on the base line supplement program.

GINGIVITIS (periodontal disease, receding gums): is the shame of the dental profession. Gingivitis is totally preventable with proper nutrition and can very frequently be cured with nutrition. It is the contention of the "orthodox" dental profession that food caught between the teeth and between the gums and tooth is the root cause of gingivitis and they have duly raised the stock worth of the dental floss companies. In reality, the reason the gums recede and food gets packed into the gingival space between the gums and tooth is that the "alveolar" bone supporting the tooth root has dissolved from a calcium deficiency and/or a phosphorus excess (i.e., too much meat, too much phosphate containing soft drinks, etc.). The alveolar bone is very thin and fragile so minute losses in bone density are reflected more severely there than, in say, the femur (thigh bone). The truth would get rid of an entire specialty of dentist so it is kept in the dental research literature. Think about it, dogs and cats don't floss and they don't get periodontal disease or receding gums unless we feed them table scraps (complete dog and cat rations have been formulated to prevent this malady) — again the veterinary profession is treating their patients better than their human counterparts!

Treatment of gingivitis includes the correction of the calcium phosphorus ratio in the diet (consider gingivitis as an osteoporosis of the jaw). The correct calcium/phosphorus ratio is 2 calcium/1 phosphorus (most American diets are 15-20 phosphorus for 1 calcium) and it is impossible to achieve without supplementation of calcium and consciously reducing the phosphorus intake (i.e., give up soft drinks, reduce meat intake, etc.). Calcium at 2,000 mg and magnesium at 1,000 mg t.i.d. with meals until teeth tighten up and gums calm down and are not so inflamed. Plant derived colloidal minerals make this aspect of prevention and treatment easy. This heavy supplementation of calcium will not cause kidney stones if you take the magnesium with it, cut back to 2,000 mg/day after the teeth tighten up. Rinse the mouth with hydrogen peroxide tooth gel and mouth wash, take vitamin C to bowel tolerance, herbs may be used for mouthwash to relieve inflammation and pain and include arnica (Arnica montana), bilberry (Vaccinium myrtillus), German chamomile (Matricaria chamomilla), high mallow (Malva Sylvestris) and tormentil bloodroot (Potentilla erecta).

GLAUCOMA: is caused by an increased pressure in the eye itself which causes a change in shape, obstructing the normal flow of fluid from the eye. Food allergies are among the most common causes of increases in eye pressure. Do the pulse test to determine if you are allergic to any foods.

Treatment of glaucoma by the "orthodox" doctor is limited to a prescription of pilocarpine 4% every 15 minutes, surgery or cortisone. You must do pulse testing and eliminate foods you are sensitive to, betaine HCl at 75-200 mg t.i.d. before meals, vitamin C to bowel tolerance, rutin at 20-50 mg t.i.d., and the base line nutritional supplement.

GLUTEN ENTEROPATHY (celiac disease): see celiac disease

GOITER (colloid goiter): is caused by a simple iodine deficiency. Nitrates are goitrogenic (stimulate goiter formation); they are found in luncheon meats, hot dogs, sausages and a variety of prepared meat products; another source of goitrogens is the nitrates in fertilizers which gets into well water — if you get your water from a farm well, have it tested for nitrates (they are carcinogenic as well as goitrogenic). Goiter is easy to diagnosis because the deficient thyroid gland enlarges 50-100 times its normal size; it is located just below the larynx in the front of the neck.

Treatment of goiter includes the removal of all goitrogens from the diet (read labels to exclude nitrates and nitrite), supplement iodine at 250 mcg/day and thyroid USP at 2-5 grains each morning, kelp is a good natural source of iodine.

GOUT (gouty arthritis): is caused by deposits of uric acid crystals in the joints and surrounding tissues. These joints, classically the great toe of each foot, are very tender and may become deformed in chronic or long-standing cases. Kidney disease and uric acid kidney stones may develop in chronic untreated cases. Elevated uric acid in the blood (above 7 mg/100 ml of serum) along with sudden onset of tender "gouty" joints is a red flag for gout.

Treatment for gout should include an avoidance of alcohol, organ meats, sea food, lentils, beans, peas and fructose sources, folic acid at 10-75 mg/day, cherries and cherry juice, herbs including gout weed (Aegopodium podagraria) and saffron (Colchicium autumnale). The "orthodox" doctors use colchicine almost exclusively as the treatment of choice, but add prednisone for inflammation.

GROWING PAINS (osgood-slaughter ox): are common in American children today; all you have to do is go to the zoo and watch parents carrying around six and seven year old children on their hip! Growing pains are totally unnecessary and are red flags for one or more nutritional deficiencies. Prevention of growing pains includes a base line nutritional supplement rich in calcium, magnesium, selenium, vitamin E and vitamin C.

Treatment of growing pains includes calcium and magnesium at 2,000 mg and 1,000 mg per day, selenium at 50-200 mcg b.i.d. and betaine HCl and pancreatic enzymes at 75-200 mg t.i.d. before meals.

GUMS (sore, pyorrhea): see gingivitis. You may also wish to rinse mouth with a tea from the root of the white pond lily (Nymphae odorata).

HAIR LOSS (alopecia): see alopecia

HANGNAILS: are caused by an essential fatty acid deficiency.

Treatment of hangnails includes flaxseed oil at 5 gm t.i.d.

and Knox gelatin at one packet daily. You may also wish to put vitamin E oil or aloe vera directly on the hangnail to soften it and reduce the probability of further tearing or infection. Small scissors or fingernail clippers can be used to "surgically" remove the skin flap.

HAY FEVER (pollen allergies): are caused by plant pollen allergies and tend to be seasonal and coincides with plant cycles. Symptoms include headache, red itchy eyes, nasal congestion and asthma.
Treatment of hay fever includes autoimmune urine therapy after the first attack each year, commercial antihistamine products (i.e., Allerest, Contac, etc.), vitamin C to bowel tolerance, bioflavonoids at 150 mg q.i.d. and rutin 50 mg t.i.d. or as needed.

HEADACHES (HA): are caused by a wide variety of problems. Food allergies (the primary cause of migraines) and hypoglycemia are major causes of headaches. Sinus headaches are often caused by allergies to pollens and milk products. Headaches can also be cyclic in PMS. Do a complete series of pulse tests and a six-hour GTT.
Treatment for headaches comes in the form of a wide variety of commercial products (i.e., aspirin, tylenol, Nuprin, Bufferin), chromium at 50-200 mcg t.i.d. betaine HCl at 75-200 mg t.i.d., avoid offending foods including all sources of caffeine, autoimmune urine therapy, vitamin C to bowel tolerance, B-3 at 450 mg time release q.i.d., B-6 at 100 mg t.i.d. or as needed, choline at 150 mg/day, flaxseed oil at 5 gm q.i.d., avoid simple carbohydrates, use proteins and amino acids for snacks, herbs including feverfew (Tanacetum parthenium), fleabane (Erigeron canadense), balm (Melissa officinalis), cowslip (Primula veris), lavender (Lavandula angustifolia),

queen-of-the-meadow (Filipendula ulmaria), valarian (Valeriana officinalis) and white willow (Salix alba).

HEARING LOSS (deafness): may require a "hearing aid" to amplify or correct the problem; on the other hand, sometimes cleaning the wax out of one's ear with hydrogen peroxide eardrops or a commercial earwax solvent will do the trick (I used to have an office down the hall from a hearing aid retailer — this fellow was so honest, he would always send his clients down the hall so I could clean their ears before he would examine them for hearing loss and fit them for hearing aids; we saw many a miracle of hearing return!!!). In children, manganese and or tin deficiency can cause reversible hearing loss; also do a pulse test for milk allergies (another common cause of deafness in kids).

HEART DISEASE (heart attack, cardiovascular disease): see cardiovascular disease; see arteriosclerosis. Prevention is the name of the game when it comes to heart disease; good nutrition means moderation in all things, no fried foods on a regular basis (to "cheat" on your program once each week is alright), the base line nutritional supplements are a must, pay special attention to essential fatty acids, avoid as much of the polyunsaturated fatty acids as you can (other than the essentials — i.e., flaxseed oil and/or salmon oil), pay special attention to selenium (500 mcg/day) and vitamin E (800-1,200 IU/day), exercise in moderation (i.e., a 30-minute walk each evening is enough), avoid vitamin D as an adult (more than 400 IU/day results in calcification of coronary arteries — the target tissue for vitamin D poisoning!). Keep a 30-minute oxygen tank in your house (a two-hour supply if you live in a rural area), learn CPR, have nitroglycerin capsules or transdermal nitroglycerin patches on hand, obtain an IV infusion set and several 500 ml bottles of lactated ringers to set up an IV should a heart attack occur (don't relegate your survival to an EMT who might get there on time — learn as much about emergency heart care as you know about your home's electrical system!!!) UNPREPAREDNESS KILLS!!!

Treatment once you have had a heart attack includes EDTA chelation (with H_2O_2 added); you may need as many as two chelations per day for 80 or more to ensure full recovery for your heart, be aggressive – your "orthodox" cardiologist will not agree to this so you will have to arrange it yourself!!! Increase your selenium intake to 1,000 mcg/day and your vitamin E to 1,200 to 2,000 IU/day, take 5-10 alfalfa tablets (Alfachlor) with each meal in addition to the base line nutrition program. Take two ounces of Oxy-Toddy in the morning when you awake and two ounces before retiring, take betaine HCl and pancreatic enzymes at 75-200 mg t.i.d. before meals. USE YOUR PDR FOR ANY MEDICATION; YOUR "ORTHODOX" CARDIOLOGIST WANTS TO PRESCRIBE FOR YOU! Don't take any medication you do not fully understand! Remember 40% of all patients are in the hospital because of iatrogenic disease (doctor mistakes in medication or surgery). Get back into your walking and/or swimming program as soon as you can.

HEARTBURN (dyspepsia, reflux): is one of the more common diseases in the USA today. Stress and aging cause a decrease in stomach acid production which allows bacteria to grow in the stomach. These opportunistic bacteria generate gas and acid that results in the "belch," "burp" and "bloat" syndrome. Prevention includes eating small meals, no fried foods, drink eight glasses of water each day to prevent constipation.

Treatment should include betaine HCl and pancreatic

enzymes at 75-200 mg t.i.d. before each meal; for acute attacks of "heartburn" includes any of the commercial products advertised on TV (i.e., R-O-L-A-I-D-S) and herbs to include peppermint (Mentha piperita) and angelica (Angelica archangelica).

HEMORRHOIDS (piles): are varicose veins in the rectum and anus that itch, bleed, become painful and eventually blocked with clots (thrombosed). The cause of hemorrhoids is primarily low fiber diets, the resulting constipation and lack of exercise. The increased pressure needed to force out a constipated bowel movement causes ballooning of the hemorrhoidal veins. Bright red blood on the toilet paper after a bowel movement is usually from an irritated hemorrhoid. You may be able to feel the large grape sized "balloon" in the hemorrhoidal vein. Prevention includes high fiber diets and exercise. Treatment of hemorrhoids includes high fiber diets (you may need to add oat bran at two heaping tbsp. in eight oz. of juice or water before bed) to encourage two bowel movements per day, hydrotherapy (Jaccuzi jet directed at hemorrhoidal tissue) b.i.d. as long as necessary, commercial topical products (i.e., Preparation H, etc.), and topical washes and/or compresses of herbs including German chamomile (Matricaria chamomilla), silver weed (Potentilla anserina), smart weed (Polygonium hydropiper), witch hazel (Hamamelis virginiana), yarrow (Achillea millefollium), juniper berries (Juniperus communis), horse chestnut (Aesculus hippocastanum) and plantain (Plantago major). SURGERY IS RARELY, IF EVER, NECESSARY!

HEPATITIS: by dictionary meaning means any inflammation of the liver, however, in daily use hepatitis refers to any of three viruses that attack the liver: 1) Hepatitis

A is transmitted by fecal - oral contamination (i.e., contaminated food, oral sex, etc.); 2) Hepatitis B is primarily transmitted by blood contamination through dirty "community" needles, hepatitis B virus causes a more severe disease and is potentially fatal; 3) Hepatitis C is a newly identified virus associated with blood transfusions that causes chronic liver disease and death. Hepatitis can appear as a minor flu-like disease to a fierce fatal liver disease depending on your immune system's ability to fight off the virus. In China, where there is an endemic hepatitis rate of 10% (that is 100 million cases a year, folks!!!) the rate of liver cancer is very high. Prevention of hepatitis is fairly simple - follow good personal hygiene, wash your hands after using the toilet, wash your hands before cooking and eating, DOCTORS AND NURSES, WASH YOUR HANDS BETWEEN PATIENTS, do not do illegal drugs, do not use "community" needles, etc. Follow the above simple rules and you will reduce your risk of contracting hepatitis by 97%. When my wife and I went to China, we took "Handi-Wipes" and washed all plates, cups and eating utensils (i.e., chopsticks, spoons, etc.) before using them, even in public restaurants — we didn't contract hepatitis. Diagnosis of hepatitis is difficult in the early stages but easy after a week or so. Loss of appetite, prostration, nausea and vomiting and fever are the early flu-like signs; after 3-10 days the urine will turn dark and jaundice (yellow eyes and skin) will appear - the patient feels better at this point. Blood test show a marked elevation in the SGOT (AST) and SGPT (ALT) up ten times the normal values; the elevated enzymes gradually decrease as recovery takes place.

Treatment of hepatitis includes bed rest, plenty of fluids including chicken soup, avoid sugar, avoid fat, avoid alcohol, vitamin B-12 at 1,000 mcg/day, folic acid at 5-10 mg/day, catechin at 1.5 gm/day, vitamin C to bowel tolerance and herbs including licorice (Glycyrrhiza glabra), chicory (Chichorium intybus) and dandelion (Taraxacum officinale), germanium at 25-50 mg/day, selenium at 200-500 mcg/day and SuperOxy Plus at one ounce on awakening and retiring.

HERPES (simplex, cold sores): is a virus that causes recurrent blisters and ulcers on the lips (Type I) and on the genitals (Type II). This disease never goes away completely (once infected, always infected); the best you can hope for is long term remission. Herpes lesions itch at the early stages and can be very painful and disfiguring. These viruses are transmitted by kissing and sexual contact. Avoid kissing and sexual activity when the lesions are active.

Treatment includes ultra violet light directly on lesion for 1-6 minutes per day, avoid high arginine foods (i.e., avoid chocolate, peanuts, nuts, seeds, grains), eat high lysine foods (i.e., meat, potatoes, milk, yeast, fish, chicken, beans, eggs), vitamin C to bowel tolerance, bioflavonoids at 200 mg t.i.d., zinc at 75 mg t.i.d., l-Lysine at 1-6 gm/day to effect, then 500 mg/day maintenance, Ribavirin at 250-500 mg/day (do not take during pregnancy) and Isoprinosin at 500-1,500 mg/day (do not take during pregnancy), and topical herb compress with walnut (Juglans nigra). There are many commercial products available for topical application.

HERPES ZOSTER (shingles): is the result of a surfacing of a long-standing infection with the "chicken pox" virus; the resultant skin eruptions are extremely painful sometimes requiring hospitalization. Extreme pain can be elicited by the touch of clothes or sheets. The path of the virus is along nerves so a regular pattern for the skin

lesions is typical.
Treatment of choice for shingles is Isoprinosin at 500-1,500 mg/day, Ribavirin at 250-500 mg/day, vitamin B-12 at 1,000 mcg/day, vitamin C to bowel tolerance, vitamin E at 800-1,200 IU/day and zinc at 75 mg t.i.d.

HIATAL HERNIA: is usually a congenital birth defect (not genetic), however, it can also be caused by crushing the chest or abdomen as in an auto accident. Gas, dyspepsia, reflux, chest pain that mimics a "heart attack" are common symptoms. It is said that more than 40% of the USA population has asymptomatic hiatal hernia by actual x-ray survey!!!
Treatment of hiatal hernia usually is restricted to treating the gas and dyspepsia. Small meals are suggested, sleeping with the head of your bed elevated often times prevents night-esophageal reflux while you sleep. When there is a large defect in the diaphragm (paraesophageal hiatal hernia) surgical repair is recommended to prevent strangulation of portions of the stomach, intestine or liver.

HICCOUGHS: are distracting and bothersome though rarely fatal. Hiccoughs are the result of spasmodic contractions of the diaphragm, closely followed by a sudden closure of the glottis. Hiccough "attacks" may be started by swallowing hot or irritating substances that irritate the nerves controlling respiration.
Treatment of hiccoughs includes holding your breath as high levels of blood carbon dioxide inhibits hiccoughs, drink a large glass of water, orange juice or lemon juice slowly, pressure on the closed eyes with the heels of your hands and digital pressure applied to the phrenic nerves just behind the sternoclavicular joint (where your collarbone joins your sternum).

HOARSENESS (laryngitis): can be caused by too much yelling as at a football game or from many of the cold and upper respiratory viruses.
Treatment of hoarseness includes use of demulcents such as slippery elm (Ulmus fulva) in lemon and honey, chickweed (Stella media) and the "singer's plant" or hedge mustard (Sisymbrium officinale) as a liquid extract.

HYPERACIDITY (stomach acid, gas): see dyspepsia. Treat with fennel tea (Foeniculum vulgare).

HYPERACTIVITY (hyperkinesis): is a very disruptive speeded up activity level to the point the attention span is less than a minute. The repetitive activity that develops is distractive to others in a classroom or family setting. Very frequently the activities are self-destructive, injurious to others and creates a learning disability. Food allergies, food sensitivities and hypoglycemia cause 95% or better of the cases of hyperactivity and hyperkinesis. Pulse testing for allergies and a six-hour GTT are essential here if you truly wish to correct the problem. Be sure to include the base line nutritional program. In addition to the behavioral problems, and certainly more insidious, are the "celiac" disease type changes in the intestines resulting from the food allergies which cause severe malabsorption of nutrients; in turn, the resultant malnutrition causes further behavioral problems.
Treatment of hyperactivity and hyperkinesis requires absolute adherence to a rotation and avoidance diet based on the results of the allergy testing and six-hour GTT; betaine HCl and pancreatic enzymes at 75-200 mg t.i.d. before meals; Feingold diet (i.e., avoid sugar, additives, food colors, etc.); IM or IV B-complex at 50 mg each per day; chromium at 25-100 mcg t.i.d. and autoimmune urine therapy.

HYPERTENSION (high blood pressure): represents an elevation of the blood pressure above 140/90 mm Hg (the upper limits of normal); either the systolic or diastolic numbers alone or both may be elevated. High blood pressure is complex and may be caused by many diseases ranging from simple nervousness in the examining room, arteriosclerosis, kidney disease and a variety of endocrine gland disorders and food allergies. Do pulse test to identify offending foods. Do a hair analysis to check for excessive heavy metals (i.e., lead, arsenic, cadmium, mercury). Don't forget the baseline nutritional supplements. CALCIUM DEFICIENT DIETS ARE KNOWN TO BE A MAJOR CAUSE OF HYPERTENSION.

Symptoms of hypertension include dizziness, red face, headache, fatigue, nosebleeds, nervousness, memory loss, edema of the optic nerve disc, strokes, etc. While not a symptom, obesity is a serious predisposing factor to hypertension.

Treatment of hypertension includes calcium (particularly useful is the plant derived colloidal minerals which are 98% absorbable), high fiber diets, rotation/avoidance diets, autoimmune urine therapy, leaning toward vegetarian diet, low fat diet, avoid sugar and refined flour, avoid more than 400 IU of vitamin D, avoid caffeinated coffee or tea, chelation with EDTA, infusions with hydrogen peroxide, flaxseed oil at 5 gm t.i.d., garlic, reduce red meat intake, consume 4-6 cups of vegetables per day, CO-Q 10 at 60 mg/day, eight glasses of water per day, lecithin at 2,500 mg t.i.d., herbs including European hawthorn (Cra-taegus oxyacantha), rauwolfia (Rauwolfia serpentina), olive (Olea europapaea). Weight loss can drop elevated blood pressure dramatically.

HYPOGLYCEMIA (low blood sugar): is placed in quotation marks in the medical literature; the "orthodox" idea for treatment of "hypoglycemia" is to "eat a candy bar anytime you feel an attack coming on" (by the way, these quotes are from the 1988 AMA Family Encyclopedia of Medicine!!!) – with such an archaic approach to the treatment of such a simple problem how can we trust the "orthodox" medical community with something as complex as cancer!!! The cause of hypoglycemia is almost always food allergies that cause a malabsorption of chromium and vanadium as a result of celiac disease type changes in the intestine and/or a large intake of purified sugar and refined flour which increases the dumping of chromium in the urine as much as 300%. The old wives tales "if you eat sugar from the sugar bowl, you will surely develop diabetes" is then quite true as untreated hypoglycemia will very frequently develop into diabetes!!! The symptoms of hypoglycemia are highly variable and may include emotional symptoms (i.e., hyperactivity, paranoia, schizophrenia, memory loss, irritability, hallucinations, depression, manic depression, dyslexia, crying, learning disabilities, etc.), sleepiness, fatigue, heart palpitations, sweating, inability to do cognitive tasks (i.e., inability to think out simple problems), explosive reactive anger, negative thinking and catatonia and/or coma-like states.

The diagnosis of hypoglycemia requires a six-hour GTT, A FASTING BLOOD SUGAR ALONE WILL NOT DIAGNOSE HYPOGLYCEMIA OR DIABETES IN 98% OF THE CASES — THERE ARE NO SHORT CUTS TO THIS DIAGNOSIS!!! A finger prick is done in the morning while fasting and the fasting blood sugar level is recorded (normal is 75 mg % give or take 5 points); 100 gm of glucose (Glucola) is ingested; a finger prick blood glucose is taken 30 minutes after ingestion and the results recorded; a finger prick blood glucose is taken at 60 minutes after ingestion of the glucose and at hourly intervals thereafter for a total of eight finger sticks (easy to remember as you have eight fingers!). It is of extreme importance to have an observer present during the entire test, not because the test is dangerous, rather because behavioral changes are best recognized by someone else. Having the "patient" write their name, draw pictures, etc. can be very useful, especially in children where they may have a difficult time describing how they feel; these tests and observations should be done every 30 minutes during the six-hour test. A chart is then developed using the numbers gathered to assess the patient's glucose status. Hypoglycemia exists when the low during the test drops below the level of the starting fasting blood sugar level. Elevated blood sugar can produce behavioral changes as the blood sugar rises after a meal much in the same way that alcohol or drugs do (in fact, many hypoglycemics are falsely accused of being intoxicated!). Diabetes can be diagnosed when the total of the results of the fasting, 30 minute, one hour and the second hour blood sugar test exceeds 600 mg % and there is sugar in the urine during the test.

Treatment of hypoglycemia includes high protein (preferably animal protein) diets as even complex carbohydrates will increase the excretion rate of chromium in the urine, simple sugars increase the excretion rate of chromium up to 300% of the normal rate!!! Chromium and vanadium are the "magic bullets" for treatment of hypoglycemia at 50-200 mcg t.i.d. with meals — THOSE INDIVIDUALS ON INSULIN SHOULD START CHROMIUM / VANADIUM THERAPY AT 25 mcg t.i.d. TO PREVENT A SUDDEN DIP IN BLOOD SUGAR; B-complex at 50 mg each t.i.d., avoid alcohol (alcohol is a simple carbohydrate); zinc at 25 mg t.i.d., and betaine HCl and pancreatic enzymes at 75-200 mg t.i.d. before meals; resolve the associated food allergies by avoidance, rotation diets and autoimmune urine therapy; ACE and other adrenal support programs are essential.

HYPOTENSION (low blood pressure): can be caused by prescribed drugs (check your PDR), heart disease, kidney disease, low blood sugar, food allergies, dehydration, adrenal exhaustion and hypothyroidism. The causative disease process must be dealt with to properly resolve hypotension. Symptoms of hypotension include low energy, dizzy feeling when you stand up fast from a lying down or sitting position, fainting, blurred vision, palpitations, inability to solve simple problems and slurring of speech.

Treatment of hypotension includes resolving the original problem, vitamin C to bowel tolerance, zinc at 50 mg t.i.d., ACE (adrenal cortical extract) sublingual, IM or IV, thyroid at 3-9 grains in the morning (too much will cause increase in heart rate and uncontrolled shaking of hands — find the OD level then back off one grain), eight glasses of water each day, acupuncture, homeopathy, reflexology, and herbs including ginseng (Panax ginseng, P. quinquefolius), rosemary (Rosmarinus officinalis) and spring adonis (Adonis vernalis).

HYPOTHYROID (low thyroid, goiter): states frequently do not produce goiter (thyroid gland enlargement), but rather produce obesity, fatigue, disinterest, low blood pressure, water retention (edema), etc. Diagnose with a basal body temperature test (take auxiliary temperature on awakening -if below 98°F, you have low thyroid).

Treatment of hypothyroidism includes thyroid at 3-9 grains each morning (excess will cause increase in heart rate and shaking of the extended arm); increase dosage to OD then back off one grain; kelp and iodine supplement at 250-500 mcg per day and herbs to include quercus marine (Fucus vesiculosis).

HYSTERIA (melancholia): is a symptomatic diagnosis. Hysteria can result from PMS, food allergies, drugs (prescribed and illegal), alcoholism, hypoglycemia, etc.). Our "orthodox" medical colleagues created the "hysterectomy" operation to resolve hysteria because of the PMS association!!! Test for food allergies (pulse test, etc.), hypoglycemia (six-hour GTT), keep a daily diary to test for PMS, use a PDR to check out any medication that you might be on.

Treatment of hysteria includes avoidance of offending foods that you might be allergic to, rotation diets, autoimmune urine therapy, essential fatty acids at 5 gm t.i.d. with meals, chromium at 50-200 mcg t.i.d. with meals, betaine HCl and pancreatic enzymes at 75-200 mg t.i.d. before meals, acupuncture, homeopathy and herbs including black hellebore (Helle-bores niger) blue cohosh (Caulophyl-lum thalictroides), mistletoe (Viscum album), B-3 at 450 mg t.i.d. (time release) and B-6 at 150-300 mg t.i.d. (take this dose for thirty days then take a 14-day break to avoid side effects).

IMMUNE DEPRESSION (immune exhaustion): is caused by a chronic process such as unrelenting stress, chronic allergies, chronic infections which result in exhaustion of the immune system and an inability to protect yourself against foreign invaders such as EBV, Candidiasis, food allergies, arthritis, cancer, etc. Anergy refers to a state in which your immune system is so exhausted that you may not react to diagnostic tests even though you have an overwhelming disease (i.e., TB, Candidiasis, etc.). DRUGS SUCH AS CORTISONE,

PREDNISONE AND CHEMOTHERAPY CAUSE IMMUNE DEPRESSION — READ YOUR PDR.
Treatment of a depressed immune system includes vitamin C to bowel tolerance, zinc at 50 mg t.i.d., vitamin A at 300,000 IU/day as beta carotene, ACE (adrenal cortical extract) sublingual, IM or EV, germanium at 50 mg orally or IM daily, acupuncture, homeopathy, herbs to include ginseng (Panax ginseng), selenium at 1,000 mcg/day and plant derived colloidal minerals.

IMMUNIZATION (vaccination): is perhaps the greatest interface between government and freedom of choice in your own health care!!! Today the government says you will vaccinate your children or they will not be admitted to school (this is the same government who says that AIDS infected children should be in public schools!!!), state governments have even gone to the extreme to say that if you don't vaccinate your children, you will be charged with child abuse and your children placed in a foster home!!! Many states are trying to eliminate the religious exemption for vaccination — VACCINATION APPEARS TO BE A BATTLEFIELD TAKING SHAPE BETWEEN THE ORTHODOX MEDICAL ADVISORS AND OUR CONSTITUTIONAL RIGHTS TO FREEDOM OF CHOICE!!! Don't forget that many vaccination programs have been the carrier for many catastrophic diseases (some experts believe that AIDS was originally spread through vaccination programs including hepatitis vaccination to homosexuals and flu and smallpox vaccines throughout Africa). DON'T FORGET THE HERBAL BOSTON TEA PARTY!!!

IMMUNOTHERAPY: is a play on words as the "orthodox" medical doctor's practice it as their approach is chemotherapy and cortisone (which actually depresses the immune system). Immunotherapy should be designed to increase the immune system's ability to cope and adjust to all invaders. The need for immunotherapy includes cancer, arthritis, food allergies, multiple sclerosis, SLE and ALS.

Treatment to provide immunotherapy includes Immu-Stim IM or capsules at 2 b.i.d., sublingual allergens for allergies, autoimmune urine therapy, avoidance of food allergens, rotation diets, vitamin C to bowel tolerance, vitamin A at 300,000 IU/day as beta carotene, zinc at 50 mg t.i.d., germanium at 50 mg/day orally or IM, selenium at 1,000 mcg/day orally, IV or IM, acupuncture, and herbs to include ginseng (Panax ginseng).

IMPETIGO (ecthyma): is a form of dermatitis in children that may take the form of blisters filled with straw colored fluid or pus or skin ulcers. Impetigo primarily affects the exposed areas of skin such as the face, arms and legs. The "orthodox" doctors believe that impetigo is caused by a Streptococcus bacteria and treat solely with antibiotics over a long period of time. It appears, though, that impetigo is more sinister than a simple infection, rather it is an early sign of immune depression which allows normal skin organisms to flourish at an unchecked rate and cause disease. Food allergies (i.e., milk, wheat, soy) are frequently the original source of the immune depression in children, on occasion contact dermatitis from detergents will be diagnosed as impetigo. Untreated impetigo can result in deep infections of the tissue beneath the skin and in the lymph nodes.

Treatment of impetigo includes topical washes with boric acid and herbs such as comfrey (Symphytum officinale), echinacea (Echinacea angustifolia) and golden seal (Hydrastis canadensis), topical or systemic penicillin may be necessary in cases where impetigo occurs on the face to prevent scaring, vitamin C to bowel tolerance, vitamin A 25,000-300,000 IU/day as beta carotene, zinc at 25-30 mg t.i.d., avoidance or rotation diets for food allergies, autoimmune urine therapy, increase animal protein level of the diet (i.e., eggs, chicken and fish).

IMPOTENCE (inability to have an erection): can be caused by wide variety of problems including an unstimulating partner, psychological domination by your partner (i.e., domineering wife syndrome), guilt (i.e., having had an extramarital affair), malnutrition of various sorts, hypothyroidism, low blood pressure, adrenal exhaustion, hypoglycemia, stress, post surgical damage (prostate surgery), etc. Solving any associated problems first will guarantee results.

Treatment of impotence should include relaxation, spend time with your mate, set up romantic situations (the interpretation of the word romantic is an individual thing — flowers excite some people and turn others off, alcohol excites some people and anesthetizes others!!!), acupuncture, homeopathy and herbs to include ginseng (Panax ginseng), nux vomica (Strychnos nux vomica), sarsapilla (Smilax officinalis), saw palmetto (Serenoa serrulata), Zumba, oral testosterone (i.e., glandular food supplements and testosterone IM) can be of value. Don't forget the base line nutrition program and include the plant derived colloidal minerals (most satisfied wives ask for it by the 55 gallon drum!). The techniques of Master and Johnson can be very useful and can be a "self-help" technique employed without the need for an expensive counselor: Step 1) nongenital pleasuring (i.e., massage, reflexology, etc.); Step 2) genital pleasuring (i.e., genital foreplay); and Step 3) nondemand lovemaking (i.e., neither the "guy" or the "doll" expects to be brought to a climax).

INCONTINENCE (inability to control bowels or bladder): can be caused by a wide variety of diseases (i.e., benign prostatic hyperplasia, MD, MS, cancer, ALS, stroke, etc.), injury (including surgery, obstetrical procedures), food allergies and hypoglycemia. Correcting the underlying diseases or injury is a must if the desired results are to be achieved.

Treatment of incontinence should include Kegel's exercises (i.e., contracting the floor of the pelvis as if trying to stop a bowel movement) at about 250-500/day, essential fatty acids at 5 gm t.i.d., selenium at 500 mcg/day, vitamin E at 800-1,200 IU/day, betaine HCl and pancreatic enzymes at 75-200 mg t.i.d. before meals, avoidance and rotation diets of offending food allergens, chromium at 25-200 mcg/day, and herbs to include saw palmetto (Serenoa serrulata) and ginseng (Panax ginseng).

INFARCTION (cerebral-stroke; heart-heart attack): is the death of an area of tissue because the blood supply was stopped by a plug or "thrombi" (i.e., blood clot, clump of tumor cells, clump of bacterial cells). If vital areas of the heart or brain are affected, the "stroke" or "heart attack" will be fatal; if nonvital areas are affected, speech, vision, muscular function and heart capacity are significantly affected until repair and/ or compensation by surrounding areas affected, the "stroke" or "heart attack" will be fatal; if nonvital areas are affected, speech, vision, muscular function and heart capacity are significantly affected until repair and/or compensation by surrounding tissue can take place. Prevention is always better than trying to "come from behind" and repair a "stroke" or "heart attack."

Treatment and repair of infarction should include vitamin C to bowel tolerance, vitamin E at 800-1,200 IU/day, selenium at 500-1,000 mcg/day orally or IM, vitamin A at 300,000 IU/day as beta carotene, chelation with EDTA, hydrogen peroxide IV, betaine HCl and pancreatic enzymes at 200-500 mg t.i.d. 15 minutes before meals . If clumps of bacteria are involved (i.e., rheumatic fever) then antibiotics (penicillin or tetracycline) will be required to resolve the current problem and prevent further damage.

INFECTION (invasion of tissues by bacteria, viruses, fungus: is caused by two factors: 1) an infective "dose" of organisms; and 2) a low state of resistance by the host. The base line nutrient program will provide the necessary "macro" and "micro" elements for maintenance and repair of the immune system; be sure to do pulse tests to determine food allergies; use common sense and reasonable precautions when in contact with individuals who have contagious diseases (i.e., measles, mumps, scarlet fever, meningitis, hepatitis, herpes simplex, herpes 2, venereal disease, flu, infectious mononucleosis, lungworm, athlete's foot, EBV, AIDS, etc.).
Treatment of infections should include the use of echinacea (Echinacea angustifolia), golden seal (Hydrastis canadensis), garlic (Allium sativum), vitamin C to bowel tolerance, vitamin A at 300,000 IU/day as beta carotene, zinc at 50 mg t.i.d., selenium at 500-1,000 mcg/day, Immu-Stim IM or orally 2 capsules b.i.d., Isoprinosin at 100-300 mg/day, Ribavirin, H_2O_2 in 250 ml infusion over four hours; antibiotics and antifungal medications are sometimes necessary in lifesaving situations.

INFERTILITY (curable inability to have children): is usually caused by a nutritional deficiency of some nutrient. We have cured several hundred cases of infertility by simple supplementation of vitamins and minerals and digestive aids. Food allergies may be involved by causing celiac disease type changes in the intestine and, thus, affecting absorption.

Treatment of infertility should include the base line nutritional program (include plant derived colloidal minerals) , resolve food allergies by avoidance and rotation diets, eat high protein diets (up to 200 gm/day), essential fatty acids at 5 gm t.i.d., 1-arginine at 500 mg t.i.d., zinc at 50 gm t.i.d., selenium at 250 mcg/day, vitamin A at 100,000 IU/day for 30 days then drop to 25,000 IU/day, germanium at 50 mg/day; acupuncture, and herbs including ginseng (Panax ginseng), leek (Allium perrum), garlic (Allium sativum).

INFLAMMATION: can result from injury, arthritis, infection, cancer. Symptoms of inflammation include swelling, tenderness, discharges, edema, fever, allergies, etc. Treatment of inflammation include DMSO, autoimmune urine therapy, proteolytic enzymes orally (i.e., chymotrypsin, pancreatic enzymes, bromelin, trypsin), vitamin C to bowel tolerance, vitamin E at 800-1,200 IU/day, zinc at 50 mg t.i.d., essential fatty acids at 5 gm t.i.d., bioflavonoids 150 mg/day, quercetin 100 mg/day, d-phenylalanine, 1-tryptophane and d1-valine each at 1.5 gm/day, acupuncture, herbs including camphor (Cinnamonum camphora), comfrey (Symphytum officinale) and feverfew (Chrysanthemum parthenium).

INDIGESTION (dyspepsia, belch, burp, and bloat): occurs as a natural course of aging, as a result of stress and overeating. In the course of aging, the stomach begins to loose its ability to produce hydrochloric acid — this process begins at about age 35. Food allergies can contribute to this syndrome. The pulse test should be

used to determine food allergies.
Treatment of indigestion should include Kaopectate or Pepto Bismol for acute diarrhea, betaine HCl and pancreatic enzymes at 75-200 mg t.i.d. before meals, mint tea as needed to calm stomach, English bitters (Gentiana lutea) before each meal, vitamin E at 800-1,200 IU/day, selenium at 500 mcg/day, calcium and magnesium at 2,000 and 1,000 mg/day, acupuncture, homeopathy, herbs such as balm (Melissa officinalis), bitter orange (Citrus aurantium), celandine (Chelidonium majus), fennel (Foeniculum vulgare), hops (Humulus lupulus), masterwort (Peucedanum ostruthium), peppermint (Mentha piperita), wormwood (Artemisia absinthium), yarrow (Achillea millefolium) and marshmallow (Althacea officinalis).

INSOMNIA (inability to sleep): can be caused by stress, excitement and drugs including caffeine (i.e., coffee, cola soft drinks, chocolate, etc.). Use your PDR if you are on prescription drugs. Food allergies and hypoglycemia can cause insomnia. Use the pulse test and six-hour GTT.
Treatment for insomnia includes avoidance of caffeine and offending food allergens, calcium (especially plant derived colloidal calcium), chromium at 25-200 mcg t.i.d., acupuncture, homeopathy, d1-phenylalanine at 250 mg t.i.d., 1-tryptophan at 1,000 mg t.i.d., inositol at 500 mg/day, niacinamide at 1,000 mg at bedtime, and herbs including valerian (Valeriana officinalis), passion flower (Passiflora incarnata), hops (Humulus lupulus) and California poppy (Eschscholzia California) and B-3 (niacin) at 450 mg t.i.d. (time release). Don't forget the base line nutrition program.

IRRITABLE BOWEL SYNDROME: will alternate between constipation and diarrhea. Food allergies are the most frequent cause of this very distressing syndrome. Small intestine damage includes celiac disease like changes, edema, ulceration and catarrhal inflammation. This "orthodox" approach to treating irritable bowel syndrome is low fiber diets, cortisone and Tagamet. The pulse test is an extremely useful test for determining the individual cause of irritable bowel syndrome.

Treatment of irritable bowel syndrome should include high fiber diets, 4-6 cups of fruit and vegetables per day, eliminate caffeine, sugar and offending foods based on the pulse test (i.e., wheat, milk, soy), betaine HCl and pancreatic enzymes at 75-200 mg t.i.d. before meals, folic acid at 5-25 mg/day, gluten free diet and eight glasses of water each day. Don't forget the base line nutrition supplement program. Herbs including marshmallow (Althaea officinalis). A macrobiotic diet can be of great benefit here.

ITCHING (pruritis): can be caused by dry skin, contact with irritants, and contact and food allergies. Pulse test and challenge tests are used to determine allergens and irritants. Resolving the basic problem is essential to eliminating itching.

Treatment (symptomatic) of itching includes the use of topical applications of Caladryl, aloe vera (Aloe spp)., salt rubs, dilute vinegar (50%), and washes with herbal compresses (see dermatitis). Oral treatment should include 5 gm flaxseed oil t.i.d., zinc 50 mg t.i.d., vitamin A at 300,000 IU/day as beta carotene. Don't forget the base line nutritional program.

JAUNDICE (icterus, yellow eyes): can be caused by blockage of the bile duct system in the liver (gallstones, tumor, hepatitis), and/or destruction of RBC's (Rh factor, blood parasites-malaria). Diagnosis is a critical problem when jaundice is present. Examining the "whites" of the eye (sclera) will reveal jaundice by the presence of a yellow coloration which is absent when the skin is yellow from a high beta carotene consumption. Blood tests will differentiate between obstruction (i.e., elevated bilirubin — above 2.0-2.5 mg %) and RBC destruction (i.e., unconjugated or indirect bilirubin are elevated).

Treatment of jaundice includes exposure to ultraviolet light to speed up elimination, liver flush (three days of apple juice followed by a cup of olive oil and a cup of lemon juice), vitamin C to bowel tolerance, vitamin A at 300,000 IU/day as beta carotene, selenium at 500-1,000 mcg/day, vitamin E at 800-1,200 IU/day, and herbs including licorice (Glycyrrhiza glabra), agrimony (Agrimonia eupatoria), celadine (Chelidonium majus), chionanthus (Chionanthus virginica).

JOINT PAIN: can be caused by a variety of disease processes including arthritis, osteoporosis, rickets, gout, obesity and various nutritional deficiencies (i.e., calcium, magnesium, sulfur, sulfur bearing amino acids and copper) and food allergies/ sensitivities.

Treatment of joint pain includes the correction of any overt or underlying disease, calcium and magnesium at 2,000 and 1,000 mg per day, cartilage at 5 gm t.i.d., gelatin (unsweetened) once per day, copper at 2-5 mg/day (a copper bracelet can be of great value), B-6 at 100 mg t.i.d., mineral bath hydrotherapy and ultra violet light exposure at 1-6 minutes, symptomatic treatment of joint pain includes pain gels, DMSO and acupuncture. Chiropractic can be of great value in treating and providing symptomatic relief of a variety of joint problems including subluxations of the spine, ribs and pelvis.

Plant derived colloidal minerals provide an exceptional source of minerals that are 98% absorbable.

KEGEL'S EXERCISE: is a great way to condition the voluntary muscles of the pelvic floor in both males and females. This exercise is useful for prenatal conditioning of the pelvic muscles, vaginal muscles, urethral muscles in both male and female for urinary incontinence and urgency. To perform the Kegel's exercise you tighten the muscles of the pelvic floor as if you were trying stop a bowel movement; you can also add the variation of stopping your urine stream at will as often as you can. Try to do several hundred each day.

KERATOMALACIA (xerophthalmia): is recognized as a hazy dry cornea (the domed clear bulge on the front of the eye) that becomes ulcerated. Symptoms include extreme dryness of the eyes with blinking in attempts to keep the eyes moist, conjunctivitis, and night blindness. Fat-like spots (Bitots spots) can be found on the "white" of the eye ball. Untreated keratomalacia can result in permanent blindness.
Treatment of keratomalacia includes vitamin A at 25,000 IU (kids) to 300,000 IU (adults) per day as beta carotene, zinc at 10-50 mg t.i.d. and increase the animal protein to 120 gm day (i.e., chicken, fish, eggs, milk, lamb, pork or beef). Don't forget the base line nutritional supplement program.

KERATOSIS: is a "goose bump" like keratin build up in the openings of the hair follicles. These pinhead sized "plugs" are found in greatest numbers on the backs of the arms, thighs and buttocks. The "orthodox" doctors claim that treatment is unnecessary, however, keratosis is, in fact, a symptom of a chronic vitamin A deficiency. Treatment of keratosis includes vitamin A at 25,000 IU (kids) to 300,000 IU (adults) per day as beta carotene, zinc at 10-50 mg. t.i.d., increase protein at 120 gms per day and don't forget the base line nutrition program.

KERNICTERUS: is the depositing of bile pigments into the brain of newborn children after an extended elevation of bilirubin (bile pigments produced from RBC breakdown). Symptoms mimic those of cerebral palsy (i.e., lethargy, poor feeding, vomiting, incoordination, seizures and death). Prevention and treatment of kernicterus includes frequent feeding of the infant to reduce absorption of bile pigments, exposure to blue and ultra violet light to photo-oxidize bilirubin (a transient lactose intolerance is associated with light therapy in infants that results in diarrhea — this does not appear to have any permanent consequences).

KETOACIDOSIS (ketosis): results from a low glucose supply to the liver which forces it to metabolize fat — the resulting by-products are "ketone bodies" (i.e., acetoacetic acid, B-hydroxyburytic acid and acetone). Ketosis occurs in diabetes, alcoholism, hypoglycemia and starvation. The breath will smell like acetone, nausea and vomiting, air hunger, confusion or coma, extreme thirst and weight loss. A positive urine "dipstick" for ketone bodies is an easy way to confirm your suspicious. Treatment of ketosis includes resolving the basic disease process (i.e., diabetes, hypoglycemia, alcoholism, starvation, etc.), increasing the complex carbohydrate intake, chromium at 50-200 mcg t.i.d. and the base line nutritional program.

KIDNEY DISEASE (kidney stones): can be caused by a variety of infections, toxins and nutritional excesses (i.e., hypervitaminosis D) and deficiencies (i.e., deficiencies of vitamin A, selenium and zinc). Kidney disease can be secondary to cardiovascular disease or diabetes. Kidney stones, contrary to popular belief by the "orthodox" doctor, are caused by calcium and magnesium deficiencies which cause a depletion of calcium from your bones which is the source of the calcium found in kidney stones. Prevention of kidney stones includes adequate levels of supplementary calcium and magnesium (impossible to get enough from your diet especially if you are a big consumer of phosphorus — meat and carbonated soft drinks). Excess vitamin D (suntanning, fish oil and supplementation) concurrently with a calcium deficiency will accelerate the depletion and, thus, increase the risk of stones. Check for cadmium toxicity with a hair analysis.

Treatment of kidney disease and kidney stones should include supplementation of calcium and magnesium at 2,000 mg and 1,000 mg per day, reduction of your phosphorus intake, adequate vitamin A nutriture at 25,000-300,000 IU vitamin A per day as beta carotene, B-6 at 50 mg t.i.d., lysine and glutamic acid and herbs including dandelion (Taraxacum officinale), dwarf elder (Sambucus ebulus), goldenrod (Solidago virgaurea), Java tea (Orthosiphon stamineus), parsley (Petro Selinum crispum), horsetail (Equisetum spp.), mugwort (Artemisia vulgaris) and cranberry juice. Chelation will help kidney disease, kidney disease that is secondary to cardiovascular disease and cadmium toxicity. An acute or sudden kidney stone blockage may require the pain relief of morphine as it can be excruciating; you may also wish to use a prednisone for three days to reduce the inflammation in the ureter (the tube from the kidney to the bladder) so that you can pass the stones. Stones lodged in the kidney can be reduced to harmless powder by a machine known as a "lithotripter" — it is an ultra sound machine that actually shatters the stones without surgery.

KORSAKOFF'S SYNDROME (recent memory loss, false Alzheimers Disease): is characterized by an inability to record new memory; the patient can perform detailed tasks learned before onset but cannot learn the simplest of new tasks. This type of "amnesia" can result from a blow to the head or be the result of chronic alcoholism and vitamin B-1 deficiency. Confabulation or producing imaginary experiences for those that cannot be recalled is a consistent feature of Korsakoff's syndrome. If the disease is the result of a blow to the head, there is a good chance of recovery, if the brain tissue has been damaged by alcoholism or vitamin B-1 deficiency, the process may be difficult to treat.

Treatment of Korsakoff's syndrome includes chelation, hydrogen peroxide IV, vitamin B-1 at 100 mg t.i.d., lecithin at 2,500 mg. t.i.d., avoid alcohol, avoid sugar, chromium/vanadium at 50-200 mcg t.i.d., betaine HCl and pancreatic enzymes at 75-200 mg t.i.d. before meals; hydergine at 4.5-9 mg/day, vasopressin (Diapid) at 12-16 units per day as a nasal spray, centrophenoxine at 4.4-8.0 gm per day and piracetam (Dinagen) at 1.6-4.8 gm per day.

KWASHIORKOR (protein starvation): is thought of as a disease of starving African children; it is classed as protein/calorie starvation and is characterized by a distended bloated belly and edema and "dropsy" because low blood protein levels can't hold water in the blood vessels so it simply "leaks" out. By now you will recognize that this happens to unschooled dieters, cancer patients, vegans and frutarians who take in less than optimal amounts of complete proteins. Don't forget the base line nutritional supplementation.

Treatment of Kwashiorkor includes adequate intake of complete animal protein (i.e., greater than 120 gms per day), a calorie intake of 3,000 calories per day, selenium at 200 mcg per day and chromium at 50-200 mcg t.i.d.

LABOR (induce): can be made easier and assisted by herbs including blue cohosh (Caulophyllus thalictroides) and raspberry tea (Rubus idaeus), corn ergot (Ustilago maydis) can be used to stop postpartum hemorrhage (orally or IM). Taking training classes (i.e., Lamaze) will help train the mother to be to relax during contractions (labor pains) and help train the "coach" to assist and how to recognize potential trouble. Home births are safer than hospital births and, in addition, the hospital rate of caesarian section is 35% (vaginal births net the "orthodox" OB/GYN $800-$1,200; caesarian sections net them $2,500!!!)

LACTATION (induce): can be induced or enhanced with herbs including milkweed (Asclepias galioides), caraway (Carum carvi), fenugreek (Trigonella foenum-graecum) and goat's rue (Galega officinalis).

LACTATION (reduce): can be reduced and breast pain of engorgement relieved by goldenrod (Solidago petradoria).

LACTASE DEFICIENCY (cow's milk sensitivity): is a form of carbohydrate intolerance that results from a deficiency of the enzyme required to breakdown milk sugar (lactose) into glucose and galactose. Lactase deficiency is characterized by bloating and diarrhea with violent abdominal cramps following the ingestion of cow's milk and cow's milk products. Lactase deficiency occurs at 20% adults of Northwest European origin, at 75% in adults of all other ethnic groups, 90% of all orientals, 75% in blacks and American Indians. The ability to digest lactose is gradually lost between the ages of 10-20 years of age.

Treatment of lactose intolerance includes avoidance of lactose containing foods and/or predigestion of lactose by adding lactase to milk containing foods.

LARYNGITIS (loss of voice): can be caused by bacterial and/or viral infections and extreme overuse of the vocal cords (i.e., yelling at a football or hockey game). Very frequently, the temperature is not elevated and voice loss is the only symptom. "Strep" throat can be a cause that can be potentially dangerous and lead to rheumatic fever or meningitis if not dealt with properly. Hoarseness, voice change or complete loss of voice (aphonia), tickling/raw throat are all symptoms.

Treatment of laryngitis can include penicillin or tetracyclines for "Strep" throat at 250 mg orally q 6 h for 10-12 days, voice rest, honey/lemon preparations and herbs including cajuput (Melaleuca leucadendron), sunflower (Helianthus annus), pine oils (Pinnus sylvestris), black caraway (Pimpinella saxifraga), garden sage (Salvia officinalis), high mallow (Malva sylvestris), wild ginger (Asarum europium), eucalyptus (Eucalyptus globulus). Viral laryngitis may be treated with Isoprinosin at 500-1,500 mg per day or Ribavirin at 250-1,500 mg per day (pregnant women should avoid these drugs as they are teratogenic in lab animals).

LAXATIVE: includes many OTC preparations such as Ex-Lax and Milk of Magnesia and herbs including senna (Cassia aqutifolia), flaxseed or flaxseed oil (Linum ustatissimum), alder buckthorn (Rhamnus fragula), cascara sagrada (Rhamnus purshiana), juniper (Juniperus communis) and manna ash (Fraxinus ornus).

LEAD POISONING (plumbism): can cause a wide variety of symptoms and syndromes including learning disabilities, kidney disease stunted bone growth, headaches and gastrointestinal disease. Very often the eating of lead is the result of "pica" or a compulsive eating of unusual things because of mineral deficiencies. Sources of lead include paint chips, window caulking, glaze from pottery, lead arsenate garden sprays, pollution from leaded fuels, inhalation of smoke from burning batteries and large lead insulated wire. Diagnosis of lead poisoning can be made from a hair analysis in chronic cases or blood in sudden onset acute cases.

Treatment of lead poisoning includes vitamin C to bowel tolerance, chelation with calcium EDTA at 10-25 infusions and/or oral D-penicillamine. Don't forget the base line nutritional supplement program containing plant derived colloidal minerals because the chelation process will tend to deplete body stores of minerals (selenium is of particular value).

LEARNING DISORDERS (dyslexia, hyperactivity, autism): see autism, dyslexia, food allergies, hypoglycemia, hyperactivity and lead poisoning.

LEGIONNAIRES' DISEASE: is caused by an infection with Legionella pneumophila; the disease is characterized by pneumophila; the disease is characterized by pneumonia, high fever, slow heart, rate, dry cough, chills pleuritis and diarrhea. Legionnaires' disease is a relatively new disease only being discovered in 1976. URI is significantly absent in this disease. Untreated Legionnaires' disease will be fatal in 80% of the cases. Diagnosis requires growing the organism on charcoal-yeast ex-

tract from sputum. Immunosuppressed patients such as chemotherapy treated cancer patients, transplant patients and AIDS patients are most susceptible.
Treatment of Legionnaires' disease is specific with erythromycin at 500 mg to 1 gm orally or IV q 6 H for three weeks.

LENTIGO-MALIGNA MELANOMA (melanoma, skin cancer): originates from the Hutchinson's freckle on sun exposed areas on the face, neck, arms and torso. These skin cancers appear as large flat, tan or brown lesions with darker black or brown spots dotted on its surface. These are slow growing cancers requiring about ten years to invade the dermis or deep skin layers.

Treatment of L-M melanoma can include excision biopsy or complete surgical removal; frequently these tumors are on the face and a cream such as Carcelim may be more desirable. Carcelim requires 30 days of application to remove the melanoma. Take vitamin C to bowel tolerance, vitamin V at 300,000 IU/day as beta carotene, selenium at 1,000 mcg per day and use a #40 sunscreen to prevent new cancers. Don't forget the base line nutritional supplement program.

LEPTOSPIROSIS (Weil's Disease, infectious jaundice): is an infectious disease caused by Leptospira spp a spirochete bacteria carried by dogs, rats and various species of wild animals. Individuals are infected by urine contaminated water, cuts while skinning or butchering infected animals. Symptoms include anemia, jaundice, proteinuria, hematuria and, on occasion, aseptic meningitis. Fever and chills are consistent symptoms. Blood tests or urine cultures are necessary for diagnosis.
Treatment with antibiotics is most effective if instituted

within four days of onset. Tetracycline at 500 mg q.i.d. is effective.

LEUKEMIA (blood cancer): is a cancer of the blood forming tissues of the bone marrow. No exact cause is proven but viruses, radiation and chemicals such as benzene are implicated. Leukemia produces a defect in the maturation process of WBCs resulting in large numbers of immature WBCs in the circulating blood. Diagnosis is made from a blood test which shows anemia, low platelets, increased lymphoblasts (immature WBC) and an elevated total WBC count. Symptoms include weakness, joint pain, anemia, enlarged lymph nodes, enlarged spleen.
Treatment includes Laetrile, hydrogen peroxide, DMSO (matures the immature cells in the circulation) IV, Onco-Tox, shark liver extract, hydrazine sulfate, cesium chloride, polyerga, germanium, carbamide and, as needed, micro-dose chemotherapy, amino acids IV, vitamin C to bowel tolerance, selenium at 500-1,000 mcg per day, and vitamin A at 300,000 IU as beta carotene.

LEUKORRHEA (vaginal discharge): is a nonspecific vaginal discharge containing mucus, WBCs and, on occasion, is tinged with blood. Leukorrhea can be caused by Candida albicans, Hemophilus vaginalis, Streptococcus spp., Staphylococcus (the bacteria that will cause toxic shock syndrome when vaginal tampons are used incorrectly) or Neisseria gonorrhoea. Culture (growth of bacteria) and/or looking at the discharge under the microscope is required for specific diagnosis.
Treatment of leukorrhea should include specific treatment for the causative organism (i.e., vaginal application of triple sulfonamide creams, oxytetracycline vaginal suppositories, vaginal douches with vinegar 30 ml/

pint of water, 1.5 % H_2O_2 as *Oxy Toddy*). Gonorrhea will require systemic antibiotics as well (please note.that any venereal disease must be reported to the Public Health Department).

LICE (pediculosis): can infest the head (Pediculus humanus capitis), body (P.h. corporis) and pubic area (Phthirius pubis). Eggs (nits) are white oval shaped seed-like objects attached to the base of the hairs; adult lice can be seen scuttling through the hair on the surface of the skin. Itching and irritated skin are the most common symptoms. Diagnosis is dependent on finding the adult lice or "nits" in the hair and scalp.

Treatment of lice includes the use of Labordor tea (Ledum latifolium) or field larkspur (Delphinium consolida) as a hair wash, use a special fine toothed comb to "harvest" the "nits;" treatment should be done daily for fourteen days to break the life cycle of the lice. For stubborn cases, you may wish to use 1% gamma benzene hexachloride daily for two days as a shampoo and reapplied in ten days (avoid prolonged use of the insecticide as it can cause genital skin irritation, especially in males).

LIFE EXPECTANCY (life span): potential for man is 120-130 years, yet the average life span based on insurance actuary tables is only 72 for males and 78 for females. This leaves a 40-50 year differential that we can work towards with hopeful expectations. The use of water filtration systems in the home, the use of air filters and conditioners for the home and work place as well as employing the base line nutrition program can add ten years to your life. The use of digestive aids (i.e., betaine HCl and pancreatic enzymes) will add an additional ten years to your life (which gives you an added twenty years when you actively and aggressively seek a healthful life.

The Hunza secret of longevity (average of 100 years with a top end of 140 years) is the daily consumption of a rich supply of plant derived colloidal minerals.
Exercise alone without attention to food allergies, digestive aids, base line nutritional supplement program, colloidal minerals and avoiding pollutants will only shorten your life and make what life you do have very sweaty!!!
Take responsibility for your own health and you will add twenty more years of life — remember that 40% of all patients in the hospital are there because of iatrogenic disease (doctor created); this fact does not deal with the number who died outside of the hospital because of mistakes in prescriptions, mistakes in diagnosis and mistakes in procedures!!!

LIVER DISEASE (cirrhosis, nonviral hepatitis): can be diagnosed by blood test showing elevation in SGOT, SGPT, GGT, alkaline phosphatase and bilirubin. Elevated ketones in the urine are clues to liver disease as well as carbohydrate metabolism Jaundice and problems with delayed clotting times and a swollen tender liver (under the ribs at the right upper quadrant), dry itchy skin (a result of problems with essential fatty acid metabolism), anemia (iron storage and B-12/folic acid) deficiencies, weight loss and ketosis are all symptoms of liver disease. ALSO SEE GALLBLADDER DISEASE.
Treatment of liver disease includes chelation with complete IV supplementation including amino acids and interlipids, vitamin C to bowel tolerance, vitamin A at 300,000 IU per day as beta carotene, B-complex at 100 mg each t.i.d., selenium at 500-1,000 mcg per day, B-12 at 1,000 mcg per day, folic acid at 15-25 mg per day, essential fatty acids (both salmon oil and flaxseed oil) at 1 gm t.i.d. and herbs including tamarac (Larix americana), parsley (Carum petroselinum), hemp acrimony

(Eupatorium cannabium) and milk thistle (Silybum marianum). Don't forget the base line nutrition program and colloidal minerals

LOCKJAW (tetanus): is caused by the toxin (waste product) of Clostridium tetani which is a normal inhabitant of animal manure. Puncture wounds contaminated by this organism cause the production of tetanus toxin which paralyzes the voluntary muscles including the jaw muscles (masseter) which gives the disease its name "lockjaw." Prevention of the infection is the best of the alternatives; squeeze the puncture wound to make it bleed; small puncture wounds of the foot or hands may require opening to allow cleaning with soap and water; follow this cleaning with disinfection with 3% hydrogen peroxide. Take cramp bark tea (Viburnum opulus) in tablespoon doses as needed. These very minimal procedures will almost 100% prevent lockjaw.

Treatment of lockjaw after it develops requires the use of tetanus neutralizing non fixed toxin, clean infected wound, disinfect wound with hydrogen peroxide, penicillin at two million u IV q 6 h or tetracycline at 500 mg IV q6 h, sedation to control muscle spasms, IV fluids and electrolytes until the patient can eat and drink on their own.

LUPUS ERYTHEMATOSUS (SLE): is considered a connective tissue disease of unknown causes; it is of interest that 90% of all cases of SLE occur in women in their 30s. The "orthodox" theory is that SLE is an "autoimmune" disease that causes the patient's own antibodies to attack themselves — the fact is the autoimmune defect occurs as a result of the disease and the presence of abnormal proteins rather than being the cause. The classical symptoms of SLE usually begin suddenly with fever, fatigue, arthritis and/or joint pain (because of this many SLE patients are misdiagnosed as having rheumatoid arthritis), a characteristic facial "butterfly" rash (typical of allergies), severe alopecia (hair loss), and papular skin lesions. Diagnosis of SLE includes recognition of a fever with the facial "butterfly" rash, poly arthritis, kidney disease, leukopenia (low WBCs), elevated blood globulins and the presence of LE cells (these only occur in 70% of SLE and are normal WBCs that have engulfed a nucleus from a destroyed cell). Do the "pulse" test to determine allergies (i.e., wheat, cow's milk and soy are the most common).

Treatment of SLE includes avoidance of offending food allergens and rotation of non allergic foods, autoimmune urine therapy, chelation with total nutrition for 15-25 infusions, essential fatty acids (salmon oil and flaxseed oil) at 5 gm t.i.d., selenium at 500-1,000 mcg per day, B-carnitine at 500 mg per day, AVOID BEEF, DAIRY AND ALFALFA. Consume daily doses of plant derived colloidal minerals.

LYME DISEASE (LD, Lyme arthritis): is a spirochete bacterial disease that is transmitted by ticks. The disease was first described in 1975 in Lyme, Connecticut thus, the name. Three to 32 days after being bitten by an infected tick a skin lesion known as an ECM (erythema chronicum migrans) will appear on the thigh, buttock or axilla. The lesion expands to a diameter of 50 cm, the lesion feels hot to the touch. There will be recurrent attacks of arthritis, fatigue, chills, fever, stiff neck, sore muscles, nausea and vomiting. Heart disease in the form of cardiomegaly and AV-block occur in 8% of the patients. Diagnosis of Lyme disease requires a high degree of awareness of the disease. Lyme disease occurs most often in children who play out in the grass or deep woods, or those who have a dog that goes out into the woods and brings home the Ixodes dammini tick. The disease occurs in clumps along the northeastern coast of the U.S., Wisconsin, California and Oregon. Patients may initially be misdiagnosed as rheumatoid arthritis, WBCs are elevated at 25,000, special blood tests are required for specific diagnosis.

Treatment of Lyme Disease requires the use of tetracycline at 250-500 mg q.i.d. for 20 days. In children where teeth are discolored by tetracyclines penicillin can be used at 20 million u/day IV in divided doses.

LYMPHOMA (cancer of the lymph nodes): see cancer

MACULAR DEGENERATION: spotty atrophy and free radical degeneration of the retina of the eye — a common cause of blindness in aging individuals, characterized by "snow" vision.

Treatment approach includes elimination of all fried foods, elimination of all sugar (natural and processed), supplement with all 90 essential nutrients (including selenium - 500 mcg.; vitamin E - 1,200 iu.; methionine) taurine 2-5 gr. and the 60 essential minerals in the plant derived colloidal form.

MALABSORPTION: see celiac disease, food allergies and hypochlorhydria

MALIGNANCY (cancer): see cancer

MALNUTRITION: can occur as an overt nutritional deficiency or secondary to extended use of medications that interfere with absorption of nutrients or malabsorption of nutrients as a result of celiac disease or hypochlorhydria. "Orthodox" doctors tend to think of malnutrition as protein/ calorie deprivation and fail to recognize macro and micro nutrient deficiencies either singly or in complex multiples, especially in their early stages. "Orthodox" doctors also fail to recognize that celiac disease changes in the small intestine lining occur as a result of "subclinical" allergies to wheat, cow's milk albumen and soy as well as other foods (i.e., rye, barley, beef, eggs, etc.).

In reality, diabetes and hypoglycemia are deficiencies of chromium and vanadium created by malabsorption as a result of celiac type changes in the small intestine; cystic fibrosis is, in reality, a deficiency of selenium and essential fatty acids brought on by celiac disease type changes in the pregnant mother and continued in the developing infant; arthritis is, in fact, a deficiency of calcium complicated by excess phosphorus in the American diet; and cancer appears to be the result of a depressed immune system that has run out of essential nutrients required to keep itself in constant repair. As wild as it seems "malnutrition" as a result of "malabsorption" appears to be the common denominator of almost all degenerative disease. Liquid plant derived colloidal minerals are the most efficient way to get minerals into malnourished humans.

MANIA (manic depression): see depression, food allergies; see hypoglycemia

MEASLES (rubeola): is a highly contagious viral disease with a sudden onset, cough, nasal drainage, conjunctivitis, Koplik's spots (eruptions on the oral and labial mucosa) and a pimple like skin rash that starts on the head and neck and spreads to the body, arms and legs. Elevated temperature to 104°F is common; pneumonia and encephalitis are unusual and potentially fatal side effects. Measles today affects young teenagers and young adults and less often infants. The incubation of measles is 7-14 days with the diagnostic Koplik's spots appearing four days after the fever starts. Having had measles gives life long immunity.

Treatment of measles should include topical OTC products to relieve itching (i.e., Caladryl), herbs including salves made of marigold (Calendula officinalis) and orally columbine (Aquilegia vulgaris), yarrow (Achillea millefolium) and pleurisy root (Asclepias tuberose).

MEASLES, GERMAN (rubella, three-day measles): is a contagious viral disease that produces mild symptoms in children including swollen lymphnodes of the head and neck. The incubation period is 14-21 days and overt symptoms may be absent in teenagers and adults. The typical skin rash occurs first on the face then spreads quickly to the body and limbs with a general body flush not unlike scarlet fever. Adults may have enlarged lymph nodes on the head and neck and adult males may complain of brief testicular pain. RUBELLA IS A DANGEROUS DISEASE IN PREGNANT WOMEN THAT CAN INDUCE SPONTANEOUS ABORTIONS AND BIRTH DEFECTS. VACCINES WILL CAUSE SIMILAR BIRTH DEFECTS AS THE DISEASE SO ARE TO BE AVOIDED DURING PREGNANCY.

Treatment for rubella is the same symptomatic therapy as that used for the nine-day measles.

MELASMA (chloasma, "mask of pregnancy"): dark brown spots with distinct margins found on the face and forehead of pregnant women and women on birth control hormones, sunlight darkens the pigment. The spots may fade after childbirth. Susceptible individuals should use sunscreens while exposed to the sun. These spots are cosmetic in nature and appear to be of no consequence to health.

MEMORY LOSS (senile dementia, Korsakoff's syndrome, Alzheimer's): can be much more devastating than a physical disability. There are a variety of causes of memory loss and it is suggested that you look up each one separately including food allergies and hypoglycemia. You should do pulse test to determine allergies or sensitivities to various foods; do a six-hour GTT to rule in or rule out hypoglycemia.
Treatment of memory loss should include avoidance of offending food allergens, avoidance of sugar, avoidance of alcohol, chromium at 25-200 mcg t.i.d., selenium at 200-1,000 mcg per day, vitamin E at 800-1,200 IU per day, B-complex at 50 mg t.i.d., Diapid (vasopressin) at 12-16 U/day (this is a nasal spray), Lucidril (centrophenoxine) at 4.4-8.0 gm/day, Dinagen (piracetam) at 1.6-4.8 gm/day (should take choline with this product) and hydergine at 9-20 mg per day.

MENARCHE (menstruation, "period"): is the regular monthly cycle of women that alternatives ovulation (mid cycle approximately at day 14) with "periods" (the 3-7 day discharge of blood and uterine lining) at the end of the cycle. "Periods" will frequently stop in women and athletes and women who drop below 20% body fat. The stopping of a period is of no health consequence in of itself but is a signal that you may be too thin for a normal cycle and ovulation. Painful "periods" are not uncommon and can be severe enough to force bed rest (this is usually the result of essential fatty acid deficiencies).
Treatment of painful or excessive menses ("heavy flow") can include OTC products (i.e., Midol) and/or herbs such as snapdragon (Linaria vulgaris), Bethroot (Trillium

erectum), black cohosh (Cimicifuga racemose), blue cohosh (Caulophyllum thalictroides), tamarac (Larix americana), alpine ragwort (Senecio fuchsii), ladies mantle (Alche milla vulgaris), St. Johns wort (Hypericum perforatum), shepherd's purse (Capsella bursa-pastoris), white deadnettle (Lamium album) and yarrow (Achillea millefolium); essential fatty acids (salmon oil and flaxseed oil) at 5 gm t.i.d., vitamin E at 800-1,200 IU/day, selenium at 500-1,000 mcg per day, iron at 25-50 mg per day (especially for vegetarian women who do not eat red meat or liver regularly).

MENINGITIS (infection of the brain and spinal cord covering): can be caused by a variety of organisms including bacteria (i.e., Neisseria meningitides, Hemophilis influenzae, Streptococcus (Diplococcus) pneumoniae, Listeria monocytogenes), fungi, and hundreds of viruses). There is great danger in this disease in that infants with meningitis often only show a fever and lethargy and there is a "blood-brain barrier" that prevents most medications from getting into the inner surface of the meninges, into the space beneath the meninges and into the brain itself. Symptoms of meningitis vary considerably but usually include a sore throat, fever, headache, stiff neck, and vomiting. Children and adults may become critically ill in 6-24 hours after the first appearance of symptoms. If you suspect meningitis, this is one disease that requires rapid diagnosis and treatment GET PATIENT TO AN EMERGENCY ROOM STAT!!! DEMAND IMMEDIATE HELP!!! Meningitis patients often die because they have waited 2-4 hours in an emergency waiting room!!!

Treatment of meningitis requires rapid diagnosis (spinal tap) and injection of antibiotics into the subdural space (under the meninges), total IV fluid and electrolyte support, and very frequently mechanical respirators — MENINGITIS IS NOT A SELF-HELP DISEASE!!!

MENINGOCELE (severe anencephlia or spina bifida): is a severe birth defect that results in exposure of the brain or spinal cord and its coverings (meninges) because of improper formation of the vertebrae. This birth defect is caused by a deficiency of folic acid, B-12, or zinc and vitamin A during early pregnancy. These deficiencies may be the result of deficient diets and/or malabsorption syndromes in the pregnant mother. Severe cases may be debilitating or fatal.
Treatment of meningocele is limited to surgery. PREVENTION is the goal here!

MENKE'S KINKY HAIR SYNDROME: is thought by the "orthodox" pediatrician to be a genetic disease, however, it appears to be a malabsorption problem in early infancy (i.e., celiac disease) that results in a copper deficiency (along with other deficiencies). It has long been known in the veterinary field that a copper deficiency causes "kinky wool" disease. Retarded growth, anemia, progressive brain degeneration, sparse brittle hair, loss of hair color, arterial aneurysms and scurvy-like bone disease (ostosis) are characteristic. Hair analysis will show very low copper levels and blood will show a low copper and low ceruloplasmin.
Treatment of Menke's syndrome includes dealing with the malabsorption problems (i.e., avoid wheat, cow's milk and soy) give copper IV at 200 ug/kg/day, give copper orally at 1-2 mg per day after relief of symptoms.

MENOPAUSE (climacteric): see climacteric

MERCURY POISONING: can result the ingestion or

inhalation of any mercurial compound and off-gassing of mercury vapors from mercury amalgam dental fillings. Symptoms include gastroenteritis, salivation, burning mouth pain, abdominal pain, nausea and vomiting, colitis, kidney disease, gingivitis, mental and emotional disturbances and nerve deficits. Multiple sclerosis is thought by many dentists and alternative health advocates to be the result of mercury poisoning. Diagnosis of mercury poisoning is easily made with a hair analysis and history of a mercury source. The mental and emotional symptoms of mercury poisoning in "hatters" in Victorian England led to the coining of the saying "as mad as a hatter" (don't forget the "mad hatter" in Alice in Wonderland).

Treatment of mercury poisoning includes the removal of the source of mercury including removing mercury amalgam dental fillings, chelation with CaEDTA (to include complete IV nutrition) and sweating (sauna) as mercury is excreted in sweat.

The use of selenium containing colloidal minerals is very effective in removing mercury from the tissues.

METABOLIC THERAPY: is the resolving or curing of disease processes by correcting the whole body metabolism through nutrition, herbs, homeopathy, acupuncture, manipulation and hydrotherapy.

METHADONE: is the drug used to facilitate opiate withdrawal. Classically methadone is given in just enough amounts to prevent the most severe withdrawal symptoms (usually 20 mg/day). The opiate (i.e., opium, morphine, etc.) withdrawal symptoms are self-limiting and not life threatening (although addicts in withdrawal often wish they were dead). The use of double the base line nutrition program for 30 days will enhance the patient's ability to get through the withdrawal — after 30 days drop to the base line nutritional supplement program and remain on it. Do pulse test to determine food sensitivities/allergies and do a six-hour GTT. Individuals addicted to drugs and/or alcohol very frequently have "addictive allergies" to food and sugar.

MIGRAINE HEADACHES: are frequently heralded by flashes of light, tingling and occurs between the ages of 10-30 years of age and more often in women than men. Nausea, vomiting, diarrhea, digital cyanosis (blue color from lack of circulation and/or oxygen), irritability and photophobia are common symptoms. "Orthodox" doctors tend to think that migraine headaches are the result of blood vessel problems; in reality, migraine attacks are the result of food allergies with the "target" tissue being the arteries which constrict in the elastic arteries in the brain and dilate the muscular scalp arteries. Do the pulse test to determine which foods you are allergic to.
Treatment and prevention are related to avoidance of food allergens which are identified by means of the pulse test, rotation diets, autoimmune urine therapy, betaine HCl and pancreatic enzymes at 75-200 mg t.i.d., vitamin C to bowel tolerance, bioflavonoids at 200 mg b.i.d. and the base line nutritional supplement program.

MISCARRIAGE (spontaneous abortion): is usually due to deficiencies of vitamins, trace minerals and/or protein. In particular, vitamin A, zinc, folic acid, selenium and complete proteins are essential to maintenance of pregnancy. Restricted diets (i.e., weight loss, incomplete vegetarian diets, incomplete rotation diets, etc.) and malabsorption syndromes (i.e., celiac disease type intestinal injury) are the most common reasons for the malnutrition that causes miscarriages and birth defects. Do the

pulse test to identify offending food allergens.
Treatment for, and prevention of, miscarriages includes the base line nutrition program for six months before attempting conception and herbs including crampbark (Viburnu-mopulus), blue cohosh (Caulophyllum thalictroides) and alfalfa.

MITRAL VALVE PROLAPSE: is a common progressive change in the left AV valve (mitral valve) and surrounding heart tissue. Most people are not aware that they have a problem, some have nonanginal chest pain, palpitations, fatigue and/or breathing problems. A late systolic "murmur" is sometimes detected when doing "squat" type exercises. If you are asymptomatic, your activities need not be restricted.
Treatment of mitral valve prolapse should include selenium at 500-1,000 mcg/day, magnesium at 1,000 mg t.i.d. and salmon oil at 1-5 gm t.i.d. and hawthorne (Crataegus oxyacantha). Don't forget the base line nutrition program. You can expect significant improvement in 30-60 days.

MONCKEBERG'S ARTERIOSCLEROSIS: is a circular calcification of the media (middle muscular/elastic layer) of small arteries. This disease is caused by hypervitaminosis D (excess vitamin D). Symptoms include hypertension and angina.
Treatment of Monkeberg's arterio sclerosis should include EDTA chelation, vitamin C to bowel tolerance, selenium at 500-1,000 mcg per day and the base line nutritional supplement program.

MONGOLISM (Down's syndrome): is a birth defect caused by a zinc deficiency in the earliest moments of conception (one third of the extra chromosome comes from the paternal parent). The "orthodox" doctors feel that mongolism is the result of a chromosomal defect that increases in risk as the maternal parent ages — it is said that women over 35 have 20% of the Down's syndrome babies (yet these women have only 6% of the babies born each year). Teenage mothers produce perhaps as many as 60% of the remaining Down's syndrome babies.

Newborn Down's syndrome babies are termed "floppy" babies as they are without muscular tone, placid and rarely cry. Physical and mental maturation is retarded and the average IQ is 50. A small head with a domed forehead is characteristic; the bridge of the nose is flattened; the eyes are slanted and have pronounced oriental folds (epicanthal folds); there are Brushfield's spots (gray salt-like grains around the outer edge of the iris) at birth, they disappear in the first year of life.

Prevention of Down's syndrome includes the base line nutritional supplement program for 90 days prior to attempting conception; test for food allergies with the pulse test to eliminate the malabsorption of zinc and other nutrients.

Treatment of Down's syndrome should include zinc at 50 mg t.i.d. and the base line nutritional supplement program; do pulse test in Down's patient to determine the presence of food allergies; avoid offending foods. You can expect an increase in IQ of 15-20 points and an improvement in physical features as long as the program is followed; withdrawal from the program results in loss of all the gains.

MORNING SICKNESS: is a nausea that occurs in the first three months of pregnancy because of rising progesterone levels. Having a complex carbohydrate or protein snack upon awakening will relieve much of the nausea; herbal tea such as dogwood (Cornus sericea) and mint (Mentha sativa); B-6 and B-complex at 25 mg t.i.d., essential fatty acids at 1,000 mg t.i.d. and the base line nutritional supplement.

MOSQUITOES: can be eliminated from your dwelling by using screen windows and doors. Electric insect "zappers" can be placed approximately 15-25 yards from the back door — the idea being that the violet light will attract the mosquitoes away from the house as well as kill a large number. In addition, to being an irritant mosquitoes carry a number of serious human diseases including meningitis, encephalitis in North America and malaria, yellow fever, meningitis and encephalitis in South America. There are numerous OTC flying insect sprays, herbs like pennyroyal (Mentha pulegium) oil rubbed on the skin and vitamins such as B-1 at 500 mg/day will also "repel" mosquitoes.

MULTIPLE SCLEROSIS (MS): is a progressive disease of the central nervous system. MS is characterized by scattered zones of demyelination (loss of the fatty insolation layer on nerves). Symptoms begin between the ages of 20-40 years and usually start with tingling and/or numbness in the arms or legs (usually "stocking" and "glove" distribution). SEE MERCURY POISONING. Weakness, clumsiness, visual problems, balance problems and dizziness and problems with bladder control follow in months or years. Knee and ankle reflexes are often increased or exaggerated. Intention tremor, nystagmus and a "scanning" speech (known as Charcot's triad) are frequent problems. Spontaneous remissions for months or years are typical of the untreated disease in the early stages. The untreated disease can be rapidly fatal in one year. Stress is known to precipitate acute attacks. Diagnosis is based on history and neurological exam (the cerebrospinal fluid is abnormal in 80% of the patients — normal CSF doesn't rule out MS). Do pulse test to determine food allergens.

Treatment offered by the "orthodox" neurologists is limited to cortisone or prednisone, unfortunately, this course of therapy is like giving aspirin to treat a brain tumor!!! It is known that avoidance of animal fats and a relatively high consumption of fish oil (cod liver oil as salmon oil) at 5 gm t.i.d. and flaxseed oil at one tbsp. b.i.d. will increase your survival rate by 50 percent; the consumption of cholesterol is of extreme importance as the myelin sheath that disappears in MS is made almost exclusively of cholesterol.

Treatment should include removal of mercury fillings, the use of CaEAP at 1 q.i.d., ., octocosanol at two capsules t.i.d., and snake venom injections daily, d-phenylalanine at 500 mg t.i.d., betaine HCl and pancreatic enzymes at 75-200 mg t.i.d., practice avoidance of known food allergens and rotation diets to heal the small intestine, avoid vitamin C supplementation (eat green vegetables and juices as a natural source of vitamin C. This treatment regime has also proved effected for ALS (Lou Gehrig's Disease),

MUMPS: is a contagious viral disease that causes painful enlargement of the salivary glands, especially the parotids. The mumps virus is very aggressive, is found in the saliva six days before the patient feels ill, found in the urine and blood. Symptoms include fever (up to 104 F), chills, the skin over the salivary glands becomes tender and shiny and edema of the parotid salivary gland that causes noticeable swelling in front of and below the ear. Complications occur in 20% or so of adult males as a painful testicular infection; testicular atrophy may follow the infection although hormone production and fertility are rarely affected.

Treatment of mumps is symptomatic including pain relief (i.e., codeine, tylenol, aspirin, etc.), bed rest, liquid diet including chicken rice soup, sugarless Jello, Gatorade, juices and herbs for symptomatic treatment including mullein (Verbascum thapsus).

MUSCULAR DYSTROPHY (MD, fibromyalgia): is another crime against the people by the "orthodox" medical doctors for reasons of money — if the total truth was shared with the public, muscular dystrophy would be totally preventable but a whole medical specialty would be wiped out!!! As crazy as this seems, look at the veterinary industry where muscle is "king" (i.e., pork chops, beef steak, lamb chops, roasts, ground red meat, chicken, turkey, etc.); muscular dystrophy has been wiped out!!! A farmer with 100 cows can expect 100 conceptions, 100 live births, 100 normal calves and 100 calves raised to market or reproductive age; how can this be that animals are treated better than people???
Prevention is the name of the game with MD; the selenium levels in preconception women is important to the maintenance of pregnancy as well as the prevention of muscular dystrophy in all of its forms (i.e., Duchenne, Erb {scapulohumerall}, Leyden-Moebius {pelvi-femoral}, Landouzy-Dejerine {facio-scapulo-humeral}, Becker's {benign juvenile} and Gowers {hands and feet}), which are in reality artificial classifications of MD by the groups of muscles initially affected. Keshan disease (heart muscular dystrophy) which is also caused by selenium deficiency should be added to the list of muscular dystrophies. In the veterinary profession, muscular dystrophy ("White Muscle Disease") has been eliminated by the use of selenium in pregnant females and rapidly growing prepubic animals. In addition to overt deficiencies of selenium in the diet, the celiac disease type changes in

the small intestine caused by food allergies is the common cause of tissue deficiencies of selenium. The symptoms of MD can start with weakness, scoliosis (curvature of the spine), enlargement of certain muscle groups (i.e., calves, trapezius, etc.) to compensate for the loss of strength of synergistic muscle groups. A muscle biopsy is usually done by a neurologist to make the diagnosis of MD. If selenium and vitamin E were to be given IM or IV at the very first onset of symptoms the disease will be arrested or cured. The "orthodox" doctors resort to prednisone and surgery!!! Death is the inevitable end for those kids with MD if they are "treated{ in the "orthodox" method — it would be much healthier to go to a veterinarian for help!!! Do the pulse test to determine food allergies and sensitivities.

Treatment of MD and/or Keshan disease includes the use of selenium orally (plant derived colloidal minerals), IV or IM at 50-1,000 mcg per day (based on weight), vitamin E IM at 80 mg per day, selenium orally at 250-1,000 mcg per day, vitamin E 800-1,200 orally, sulfur amino acids IV as a complete amino acid infusion and orally in the form of free amino acids and sugarless Jello; essential fatty acids 5 gm t.i.d., avoid food allergens, avoid excessive fats (no more than 20% of the calories each day as fat), choline as soy lecithin at 10-20 gm per day, avoid exercise for one month during initial treatment period (this is the opposite recommendation from the "orthodox" treatment) to avoid undue injury to already biochemically compromised muscle tissue.

MUSCLE CRAMPS (Charley horse): are a "mini" convulsion that is taking place in the muscle as a result of deficiencies of calcium, magnesium, potassium, selenium and/or vitamin E. Muscle cramps may be as subtle as the twitch of an eyelid, muscle flutter in arms or legs

(fasciculations) to and including the hard cramps of the feet, calves, back and neck muscles. Prevention includes the base line nutritional supplement program. Do pulse test to determine food allergies that might cause celiac disease type changes and the resultant malabsorption. Do a hair analysis to determine mineral status.
Treatment of muscle cramps can include liquid colloidal calcium, magnesium and potassium; betaine HCl and pancreatic enzymes at 75-200 mg t.i.d. before meals.

NASAL CATARRH (runny nose, stuffy nose): can be caused by a wide variety of upper respiratory viral infections. Treatment includes Contac at 1 q 12 h, cayenne pepper (Capsicum minimum), eucalyptus (Eucalyptus globulus), German chamomile (Matricaria chamomilla) and scotch pine (Pinus sylvestris).

NAUSEA: can be caused by a wide variety of diseases and syndromes ranging from nutritional deficiencies, pregnancy, hepatitis, food allergies to cancer; therefore, if nausea is a recurring problem detailed investigation should be pursued.
Treatment of nausea can include Pepto Bismol, Kaopectate, and herbs to include artichoke (Cynara scolymus), avens (Geum urbanum) and peppermint (Mentha piperita).

NERVOUS HEART (rapid beat or palpitations when nervous): tends to be common in senior citizens. Many of these cardiac symptoms are the result of B-1 (Beri-Beri) deficiencies, anemia and deficiencies of stomach acid. Do pulse test to determine if food allergies are a contributing factor.
Treatment of "nervous" heart conditions should include B-1 at 100 mg t.i.d., iron at 45-100 mg, improve general

diet, don't forget the base line nutritional supplement program and herbs including hawthorn (Crataegus oxyacantha), hops (Humulus lupulus), lavender (Lavandula angustifolia), motherwort (Leonurus cardiaca) and valerian (Valeriana officinalis); avoid offending food allergens and employ rotation diets.

NERVOUS TENSION (nervous head-aches): are usually brought on by tension and overwork; there may be a precipitating food allergy involved so don't forget to do a pulse test. Treatment includes avoidance of sugar, caffeine, food allergens, avoidance and/or reduction of stress and tension; exercise, homeopathy, acupuncture, color therapy, subliminal relaxation tapes and herbs including balm (Melissa officinalis), bitter orange (Citrus aurantium), sweet woodruff (Gallium odoraturm), wild celery (Apium graveolens) and lily-of-the valley (Convallaria magalis).

NEURALGIA (Bell's palsy, neuropathy): is an irritation of a nerve which can be caused by many diseases ranging from trauma, nutritional deficiencies (i.e., B-12, folic acid, B-1, B-6, etc.), infections (i.e., herpes, shingles, etc.), alcoholism, diabetes, MS, etc. Treatment requires attention to any and all underlying conditions; treatment of neuralgia should also include B-complex 50 t.i.d., B-12 1,000 mcg per day, essential fatty acids as EPA at 5 gm t.i.d. and flaxseed oil at one tbsp. b.i.d., calcium and magnesium at 2,000 mg and 1,000 mg per day, Isoprinosin at 500-1,500 mg/day and Ribavirin at 250-1,500 mg/day for viral neuralgias (i.e., herpes and shingles), acupuncture and herbs including lavender (Lavandula angustifolia), oats (Avena satifa), rosemary (Rosmarinus officinalis), St. Johns wort (Hypericum perforatum), white willow (Salix alba).

NIGHT BLINDNESS (xerophthalmia): is caused by a vitamin A deficiency which can be overt dietary deficiency, fat malabsorption syndrome (vitamin A is fat soluble), zinc deficiency which results in poor conversion of carotene to vitamin A by the liver; cystic fibrosis, celiac disease and various food allergies result in intestinal changes that prevent absorption of fat soluble vitamins (i.e., vitamin A, vitamin E, vitamin D and vitamin K) as well as essential fatty acids. Symptoms of night blindness include delayed adaption or complete failure of adaption to darkness. Treatment of night blindness is very specific with 25,000-300,000 IU of vitamin A per day as beta carotene and zinc at 15-50 mg t.i.d.

NIGHT TERRORS (nightmares): are almost always caused by food allergies and hypoglycemia. The pulse test and the six-hour GTT are necessary to determine the exact cause of night terrors. Remember the low point of blood sugar levels occur at 4-4 1/2 hours after consumption of food (especially sugar foods and drinks) so night terrors will occur four hours after consumption of food (especially sugar foods and drinks) so night terrors will occur four hours after consumption of "bedtime snacks" (i.e., cookies and milk). Bedwetting in children often accompanies night terrors and are the direct result of food allergies (usually milk) and hypoglycemia (sugar bedtime snacks). Treatment of night terrors includes avoidance of offending food allergens, avoidance of sugar, chromium at 25-200 mcg t.i.d., high animal protein diets, base line nutritional supplement program, avoid caffeine.

NOSEBLEEDS (epistaxis): are usually the result of vitamin K and/or vitamin C deficiencies. "Orthodox"

EENTs like to do "minor" surgery on noses to cauterize (i.e., burn) capillaries in the nasal membranes to stop the nosebleeds. Treatment for nosebleeds should include increased consumption of green leafy vegetables, reseed colon with Lactobacillus acidophilus (the bacteria will synthesize vitamin K), vitamin C to bowel tolerance, calcium and magnesium at 2,000 mg and 1,000 mg per day, vitamin E at 800-1,200 IU per day, alfalfa tablets at 5 t.i.d. with meals and herbs including toad flax (Linaria vulgaris).

NUMBNESS (tingling both hands, Carpal Tunnel Syndrome): can be caused by neuralgia (diabetes, B-12 deficiency), circulation problems and "carpal tunnel" syndrome; on occasion food allergies can cause numbness and tingling and should be considered in your diagnostic process; don't forget the possibility of MS. "Tinnel's sign" (tap wrist) with the finger to elicit pain. "Orthodox" neurologist love to do carpal tunnel surgery for this problem. Treatment for numbness and tingling should include aggressive diagnosis and treatment of any underlying condition as well as B-12 at 1000 mcg per day, B-6 at 200-300 mg t.i.d., calcium and magnesium at 2,000 mg and 1,000 mg per day and zinc at 50 mg t.i.d., B-12 at 1,000 mcg/day and colloidal minerals.

OBESITY (overweight): is a problem to various degrees in all industrialized nations and, in particular, the United States. Obesity has various causes and combinations of causes; obesity is not a simple problem. Rendered down to its simplest terms obesity is consuming and storing more calories than you are using. Starvation only complicates the correction of the problem as a starving body will shut off calorie consumption as an energy conservation move; to avoid this body maneuver, be sure to consume at least 1,000 calories per day (a gradual but permanent loss of pounds and inches will occur). Moderate exercise in the form of walking, tennis, golf, swimming and/or low impact aerobics (i.e., Chi Gong) is adequate; don't forget the base line nutritional supplements as your need for nutritional supplementation becomes critical when you are on a restricted diet. In fact 90% of obese people over eat and binge because empty calorie diets result in "pica" — a nibbling behavior caused by the bodies search for trace minerals! (Use colloidal minerals)! Test for food allergies with the pulse test and do a six-hour glucose tolerance test to determine if you have hypoglycemia or diabetes (remember a single fasting blood glucose test will miss 99.9% of all hypoglycemics and 85% of all diabetics).

"Treatment" of obesity is, in fact, a change in life style and habits requiring as complete a commitment as that required to stop smoking. Avoid offending food allergens, avoid sugar in all forms (i.e., solids as well as liquids), avoid caffeine (caffeine lowers blood sugar and makes you hungry!!!), avoid carbonated soft drinks (even the one calorie varieties are loaded with phosphates which will cause osteoporosis over the long haul — you are already on a restricted diet, don't compromise your mineral status any further); drink filtered spring water (distilled water is "hungry" water and will demineralize your bones over a long period of usage), drink 8-10 glasses of water each day (40% of your water normally comes from food — it only makes sense if you restrict your food, you will also restrict water unless you make a conscious effort to drink enough) as "compulsive" trips to the refrigerator are most often subliminal searches for water (especially right after meals), use special salts to flavor meals (potassium salt with kelp is excellent), DO NOT SKIP MEALS, make breakfast your largest most complete meal, lunch should be a moderate meal with animal protein and dinner should be a light "soup and salad," take salmon oil at 5 gm t.i.d. with meals, flaxseed oil at one tbsp. b.i.d., two heaping tbsp. of nutritional fiber in an eight ounce glass of water before bed, glucomannan at 1 gm in eight ounces of water one hour before meals, betaine HCl and pancreatic enzymes at 75-200 mg t.i.d. 15 minutes before meals and take thyroid starting at 1-3 grains (too much will make you a little jittery and increase your heart rate as much as 10-20 beats/minute — adjust up or down in dosage as needed — if you get above six grains before you OD on thyroid, you have celiac disease type because of your intestine — do pulse test and avoid allergens!!!), take herbal laxatives and/or herbal diuretic teas as necessary, subliminal weight loss tapes can be very helpful (especially at the beginning). THIS PROGRAM IS VERY COMPLEX TO BEGIN WITH — CHANGE ALL OF THE FOOD IN YOUR HOUSE — AFTER YOU REACH YOUR WEIGHT GOALS, YOU CAN SIMPLIFY YOUR WEIGHT LOSS PROGRAM.

OBSTRUCTION OF AIRWAYS (choking): will be heralded by the "universal choking sign" of both hands clutched at the throat and a loss of the ability to speak. This happens very frequently in restaurants and is often referred to as a "restaurant coronary" as most observers think the patient is having a "heart attack." Prevention includes the stopping of talking while you are chewing and swallowing food (especially meat and firm raw vegetables such as carrots and beets). Treatment of choking includes: 1) putting your finger into the back of the throat and manually removing the obstruction; 2) performing a "Heimlich" maneuver (standing behind the patient, lock your arms around them with hands locked just below the xiphoid cartilage and suddenly thrust/squeeze; for babies use hands only). If the obstruction is lodged and cannot be coughed out with the Heimlich maneuver; a tracheotomy must be performed as a lifesaving maneuver (the EMTs will not get there in time!) and you must use whatever is available (i.e., pocket knife, steak knife, etc.). The location of the incision is half way between the base of the larynx (voice box) and the notch where the collar bones join the breast bone — it must be dead center and large enough to accommodate the empty barrel of a ball point pen which will provide enough airflow for survival — the EMTs will arrive about five minutes after you have completed your "surgery," however, the patient would have died if you waited for them. If the patient's heart has also stopped as a result of the choking, you will have to perform CPR after you have created the airway.

OLIGOSPERMIA (low sperm count): is usually the result of nutritional deficiencies and/or malabsorption syndromes. Do a pulse test to determine if food allergies and celiac type changes are a factor. Infertility if the usual "red flag" that raises the question of sperm count. Place one drop of a semen sample on a slide with a cover slip on top; at high power, the live sperm should be highly motile and appear as swirling waves as "battalions" of Chinese infantry.

Treatment for oligospermia includes avoidance of offending food allergens, double the base line nutritional supplementation for 30-60 days, acupuncture, and herbs including ginseng (Panax ginseng) and herbal combinations such as Zumba.

OMPHALOCELE (umbilical hernia): is a birth defect characterized by a grape to basketball sized skin sac in the "belly button" that is lined with peritoneum (membrane lining of the abdominal cavity); the sac may contain fat and/or intestinal loops that can be pushed back into the abdominal cavity. This is a common birth defect that is caused by maternal deficiencies (and, thus, fetal deficiencies) of vitamin A and/or zinc.

Treatment of umbilical hernia requires surgery to repair the belly wall defect if the "hernial ring" (defect in the belly wall) is larger than your finger tip. If the defect is approximately the diameter of your finger tip you can heal this one at home without surgery. The technique is to place a golf ball sized ball of virgin wool on the hernia and tape it firmly down to the level of the skin. Three times each day, remove the wool ball and be sure the fat is pushed back into the belly cavity with the finger tip; at the same time, rub the "hernial ring" in a rotary fashion for several minutes to irritate it. Over a period of weeks to months, the defect will fill in and completely heal without surgery.

ORGANIC BRAIN SYNDROME (pellagra, alcoholism, dementia, depression, hyperkinesis, hypoglycemia, diabetes, PMS, paranoia, schizophrenia and learning disabilities): is caused by a wide variety of nutritional deficiencies (i.e., niacin, B-1, B-12, folic acid, chromium, etc.) and toxicities (i.e., alcoholism, lead poisoning, mercury poisoning-dental amalgam). Do a pulse test to determine if food allergies are a part of the syndromes and do a six-hour GTT to rule in or rule out diabetes or hypoglycemia (remember a single fasting blood glucose will miss 99.9% of the hypoglycemia and 85% of the diabetes). Treatment of organic mental disorders requires serious dedication to identify the underlying problems and dealing with them.

Treatment should include avoidance of food allergens,

rotation diets, betaine HCl and pancreatic enzymes at 75-200 mg. t.i.d. 15 minutes before meals, B-3 (niacin) at 450 mg t.i.d. as time release tablets, essential fatty acids as salmon and flaxseed oils at 5 mg each t.i.d., chromium at 25-200 mcg t.i.d. and zinc at 50 mg t.i.d. Don't forget the base line nutritional supplement program.

ORNITHOSIS (parrot fever): is an infectious disease caused by (Chlamydia psittaci); parrot fever is transmitted by inhaling the contaminated dust from feathers, cage bedding or feces of infected birds (i.e., parrots, parakeets, love birds and canaries or pigeons). Parrot fever is characterized by an "atypical pneumonia." Symptoms of "parrot fever" include fever, chills, weakness, loss of appetite, dry coughing initially that develops into a productive cough. At first, "parrot fever" may be diagnosed as "flu" or confused with Legionnaires disease or Q fever. Exposure to birds (especially sick ones) will offer a clue that Sherlock Holmes wouldn't miss!!! A blood test is required for specific diagnosis.

Treatment of "parrot fever" includes the use of tetracycline orally at 250-500 mg q.i.d. for 10-14 days; the cough should be controlled with codeine and strict bed rest should be enforced as untreated and uncontrolled "parrot fever" can be fatal.

OSTEOARTHRITIS (degenerative arthritis): see arthritis

OSTEITIS FIBROSA (nutritional secondary hyperparathyroidism): is also known as Paget's Disease. This is a bone disease that affects men more often than women (women get osteoporosis more frequently) and is characterized by a loss of hard bone which is replaced by fibrous connective tissue. The first signs of Paget's

Disease occur in the dental arcade by separating the teeth and loss of teeth because of loss of jaw bone. The weight bearing bones of the pelvis, femur and tibia are next; very frequently there is a loss of stature as the bones undergo rearchitecturing and kyphosis ("dowagers' hump). The cause is thought to be unknown by the "orthodox" doctors, however, in animals the cause is a reversed calcium/phosphorus dietary ratio intake in the presence of relatively large amounts of vitamin D (makes sense as men tend to be out in the sun without their shirts more often than women). Diagnosis of Paget's Disease can be made by x ray of the teeth in the earliest stages and x ray of the weight bearing bones in the more advanced stages. The blood shows an elevated alkaline phosphatase (calcium and phosphorus are usually in the normal range) and an elevated parathyroid gland hormone. (It is interesting to note that "orthodox" orthopedic doctors think of Paget's Disease as a viral infection). Treatment of Paget's Disease should include a vigorous effort to correct the dietary calcium/phosphorus ratio, reduce or eliminate red meat intake, avoid phosphate containing soft drinks, avoid all phosphate containing supplements, reduce vitamin D intake and exposure (i.e., hats, long sleeve shirts, etc.), increase calcium and magnesium intake to 2,000 mg and 1,000 mg per day, take betaine HCl and pancreatic enzymes at 75-200 mg t.i.d. 15 minutes before meals and don't forget the base line nutritional supplement program.

OSTEOPOROSIS: is a decrease in bone that usually occurs in older individuals (more frequently in women). The big push by the "orthodox" doctors is for estrogen and fluoride supplementation, yet these two compounds alone do not solve the problem. In our personal experience osteoporosis is easy to prevent and cure with proper supplementation of stomach acid (HCl) and calcium. Do a pulse test to identify any food allergens that might be causing a celiac disease type change and malabsorption syndromes. The symptoms of osteoporosis are characterized by bone pain, joint pain, "dowagers" hump and "spontaneous" fractures. Osteoporosis is the 12th most frequent cause of death in adults (following fractured hips, etc.).

Treatment of osteoporosis should include betaine HCl and pancreatic enzymes at 75-200 mg t.i.d. 15 minutes before meals, calcium and magnesium at 2,000 mg and 1,000 mg per day (or more for the first 30 days). Estrogen may be contraindicated because of the potential carcinogenic effect (known to cause breast and uterine cancer). Don't forget the plant derived colloidal minerals that include calcium, magnesium and boron.

OTITIS (earache): is an inflammation of the inner parts of the ear (externa involves the outside of the eardrum and the ear canal and interna involves the inside of the eardrum and the eustachian tube). The "orthodox" EENT approach is to give antibiotic eardrops and oral antibiotics in acute cases and to insert "tubes" into the eardrum to relieve pain in chronic cases. In reality, 95% of all otitis (earaches) is the result of a milk allergy. Do a pulse test before the eardrums are pierced and weakened unnecessarily. Milk allergies will cause a severe fever, painful earaches and burst eardrums if not corrected. Treatment of otitis should include the use of hydrogen peroxide or mullein eardrops to help relieve local inflammation, avoid cow's milk in all forms and be sure to take the base line nutritional supplement program. Aspirin or tylenol may be necessary for pain relief. Antibiotics are only justified when a Streptococcal sore throat or internal otitis is cultured.

PAIN: is caused by any abnormal process that changes the architecture of bone or soft tissue. Repairing or correcting the disease process will usually eliminate the pain without the continued need for pain medication. Treatment for pain necessarily must include an aggressive correction of any underlying disease process. Treatment of pain may include TENS (electronic pain masking), codeine, tylenol-3, aspirin with codeine, aspirin, tylenol, DMSO, acupuncture, hydrotherapy, chiropractic, and herbs including aconite (Aconitum napellus), comfrey (Symphytum officinale), chicory (Cichorium intybus) and English mandrake (Tamus communis). Don't forget plant derived colloidal minerals here.

PALPITATIONS (irregular heartbeat): can be the result of organic heart disease (this is easily determined by an EKG or ECG), food allergies (i.e., Chinese Restaurant Syndrome or allergy to MSG), nutritional deficiencies (i.e., B-1, B-3, selenium, potassium, etc.) and/or hypoglycemia.

Treatment of palpitations should include EDTA chelation for cardiovascular disease, IV hydrogen peroxide, avoid caffeine, avoid offending food allergens, avoid sugar and processed foods in all forms, vitamin B-1 at 100 mg t.i.d., B-3 at 450 mg t.i.d. as time release tablets, vitamin C to bowel tolerance and base line nutritional supplementation program; herbs including English hawthorn (Crataegus oxyacantha), lily-of-the-valley (Convallaria mejalis), hops (Humulus lupulus), lavender (Lavandula angustifolia), mother wort (Leonuruscardiaca), valerian (Valeriana officinalis) and foxglove (Digitalis purpurea).

PARASITES (worms): include a variety of roundworms (i.e., ascaris, hookworms, pinworms and whipworms), tapeworms and microscopic one cell organisms (i.e., amoeba, flagellates). Symptoms of parasites include diarrhea, abdominal pain, weight loss, anal itching, weakness and B-12 deficiency (tapeworm). Diagnosis of parasites includes a microscopic fecal exam (see laboratory section) for all intestinal parasites except for pinworms which require a Scotch tape test (see laboratory section). Treatment for parasites includes garlic (Allium sativum), peach (Prunus persica) and walnut (Juglans nigra); with heavy infestations where stronger medication is required Pyrantel pamoate (roundworms), Niclosamide (tapeworms) and Metronidazole (protozoa) should be employed.

PARKINSONISM (shaking palsy): is caused by a degeneration of the basal ganglia of the brain; symptoms are relentlessly progressive and include muscular rigidity, lack of purposeful movement, tremor and "pill rolling" tremors of the thumb and index finger. The cause of true Parkinson's Disease is unknown, however, there are numerous medications that will cause Parkinsonism-like symptoms (i.e., phenothiazines, haloperidol, reserpine) as well as carbon monoxide poisoning and excessive manganese supplementation.

Treatment of drug induced Parkinsonism should include the elimination of the offending drug ("orthodox" neurologist will usually recommend an additional drug to deal with the symptoms of the offending drug), take octacosanol at 300 mcg t.i.d., Neuro-Gen, leucine 10 gm/day, 1-methionine at 5 gm/day, essential fatty acids at one tbsp. b.i.d., 1-tyrosine at 100 mg/day, d1-phenoalanine at 100 mg t.i.d., B-1 at 200 mg t.i.d., B-6 at 100 mg t.i.d., betaine HCl and pancreatic enzymes at 75-200 mg t.i.d. before meals, and the base line nutritional supplement program; the "orthodox" neurologist treats with 1-Dopa and carbidopa which aggravates and speeds up the progress of Parkinson's Disease in a significant number of cases and has no beneficial effect in more than 50% of the cases.

PEPTIC ULCER (gastric ulcer): are thought to be caused by stress, deficiency of "vitamin U" and/or dyspepsia, in reality are caused by an infection with *Helicobacter pylori*. Symptoms of peptic ulcer include burning stomach pain, dyspepsia and weight loss. "Coffee ground" stool indicates that the ulcer is bleeding and that the patient is in eminent danger of bleeding to death. (GO TO A HOSPITAL IMMEDIATELY!) Treatment of peptic ulcer should include alfalfa (Medicago sativa) which is thought to be the richest source of "vitamin U" at ten tablets t.i.d. with meals, cabbage juice (Brassica oleracea), flax (Linum usitatissimum), German chamomile (Matricaria chamomilla) and licorice (Glycyrrhiza glabra). A 98% chance of a cure can be affected with antibiotics and bismuth every day for 4-6 weeks.

PERIODONTAL DISEASE (receding gums, pyorrhea, gingivitis): is thought by "orthodox" dentist to be caused by food particles packing into the space between teeth and between teeth and gums. In reality, all forms of periodontal disease are the result of bone loss under the gums which causes the gums to recede and allow food to pack into the space created. Again, this disease has been eliminated by the veterinary profession as a result of nutritional investigations for better health and production of pet and farm animals. I have not seen too many cows, horses, dogs and cats (nor wolves, giraffe or elephants for that matter) floss, brush their teeth or use mouthwash with fluoride. The reason that this simple concept has not been shared with the public is money!!!

Think about the toothpaste, toothbrush and floss companies that get the approval of the American Dental Association; does it not seem odd that these same companies give large grants to the dental schools (Sherlock Holmes, and maybe some union stewards, would call this one a "sweetheart deal!!!"). This appears to be another case of letting the fox "guard" the chicken house. Treatment of periodontal disease should include a correction of the dietary calcium/phosphorus ratio (i.e., give up phosphate containing soft drinks, reduce red meat consumption, reduce phytate intake (raw vegetables), supplement calcium at 2,000 mg per day and magnesium at 1,000 mg per day, remember the base line nutrition supplement program including plant derived colloidal minerals, vitamin A at 300,000 IU per day as beta carotene, vitamin C to bowel tolerance, zinc at 50 mg t.i.d., betaine HCl and pancreatic enzymes at 75-200 mg t.i.d. 15 minutes before meals, avoid sugar; use herbal and hydrogen peroxide mouthwashes and dental floss to keep teeth clean.

PHLEBITIS (varicose veins): is most common in the hemorrhoidal veins and veins of the legs. Constipation and static vertical position are the primary causative factors. Treatment of phlebitis should include consumption of eight glasses of water, two heaping tbsp. of nutritional fiber in a glass of water at bedtime, vitamin E at 800-1,200 IU/day, B-complex at 50 mg each t.i.d., vitamin C to bowel tolerance, copper at 2 gm per day, essential fatty acids at 5 gm t.i.d., and herbs including arnica (Arnica montana), comfrey (Symphytum officinale), rue (Ruta graveolens), yellow sweet clover (Melilotus officinalis) and cascara sagrada (Rhamnus purshianus).

PICA (craves dirt or paint): is a symptom of one or more nutritional deficiencies. Adults often crave ice, children eat dirt and/or paint (the latter is extremely dangerous as many paints contain lead or cadmium). A hair analysis will be invaluable to determine the patient's mineral status. Do a pulse test to determine if a celiac disease type malabsorption problem exists.

Treatment for pica should include the base line nutritional program including plant derived colloidal minerals; EDTA chelation therapy may be necessary if hair analysis shows elevated levels of lead or cadmium.

PILES (hemorrhoids): see hemorrhoids

PILONIDAL CYST: is a midline congenital defect (zinc or vitamin A, folic acid deficiency) in the sacral area. The pit often contains hair. The tract is usually asymptomatic unless it becomes plugged and becomes a cyst. Treatment of the pilonidal cyst should include a poultice of plantain (Plantago major), comfrey (Symphytum officinale) or boric acid b.i.d. until cyst opens up; on rare occasions surgical opening of the cyst is required; local anesthesia and a scalpel blade are all that is required for this relatively minor surgery.

PIMPLES (acne): see acne

PREMENSTRUAL SYNDROME (PMS, hysteria): has a long history in "orthodox" medicine.

Historically the treatment was hysterectomy (derived from hysteria) since removal of the ovaries and uterus "cured" all of the cyclical emotional symptoms leaving a precipitous menopause which could be palliated with estrogen. It is now known that deficiencies of essential fatty acids in concert with the cyclical hormone patterns of the women produce the classical PMS picture of fragile emotions, irrational behavior, mania, depression and debilitating pelvic "cramps."

Treatment of PMS includes 100 mg B-6 q 4 d, essential fatty acids at 5 mg t.i.d., vitamin A at 300,000 IU per day as beta carotene during the last 14 days of the cycle, vitamin E at 800-1,200 IU/day, calcium (especially plant derived colloidal sources) and herbs including mistletoe (Viscum album), black cohosh (Cimicifuga racemosa) and blue cohosh (Caulophyllus thalictroides).

POISON IVY: causes a contact papular dermatitis that produces a severe itch. Treatment of poison ivy dermatitis includes topical application of Caladryl, aloe vera, poultices of Solomon's seal (Polygonatum multiflorum), golden seal (Hydrastis canadensis) and plantain (Plantago major).

POOR CIRCULATION: can be caused by cardiovascular disease, low thyroid and vitamin E deficiency. Symptoms include cold hands and feet and numb tingling fingers and toes.

Treatment of poor circulation includes EDTA chelation, hydrogen peroxide IV, vitamin C to bowel tolerance, vitamin E at 800-1,200 IU/day, massage, hydrotherapy, acupuncture and herbs including ginkgo (Ginkgo biloba), hawthorn (Crataegus oxyacantha), horsetail (Equisetum arvense), lavender (Lavandula angustifolia), lily-of-the-valley (Convallaria majalis), rosemary (Rosmarinus officinalis), scotch pine (Pinus sylvestris) and cayenne pepper (Capsicum minimum).

POX (chicken pox): see chicken pox

POST PARTUM HEMORRHAGE: is the result of an atonic uterus that failed to contract hard enough, long enough allowing the open vessels to leak blood (on occasion a piece of afterbirth will remain in the uterine lining and is the source of the bleeding.

Treatment of post partum hemorrhage should include firm digital pressure on the fundus of the uterus to stimulate contraction; the use of ergot (Claviceps purpurea) orally at 10-20 minims or by injection will add sufficient contraction power.

PREGNANCY LABOR (labor): can be enhanced by the use of herbs including raspberry (Rubus idaeus) and blue cohosh (Caulophyllum thalictroides).

PREGNANCY TOXEMIA (eclampsia): is the result of low protein, low salt diets entered into an attempt to prevent excess weight gain in pregnancy. The first thoughts of restriction of weight gain occurred at the turn of the century when "orthodox" OB/GYN practitioners learned that low birth weight babies could be delivered faster and, thus, allow more calls in one day. Symptoms of preeclampsia include sudden weight gain (because of fluid accumulation as a result of low blood protein), high blood pressure, albumi-nuria; eclampsia includes the symptoms of preeclampsia plus convulsions and/or coma; both preeclampsia and eclampsia characteristically occur after the 20th week of pregnancy. The current "orthodox" treatment is hospitalization, watch until convulsions occur then give barbiturates. Treatment of preeclampsia should include a high animal protein meal plan (150 gm or more whereas the RDA is 40 gm), do not restrict salt, B-6 at 100 mg per day (drop to 50 mg per at parturition (birth) if you plan to breast freed as high levels of B-6 will reduce production of breast milk), base line nutritional supplement program and 10-12 glasses of water and/or juice per day, especially in the warm summer months.

PROSTATE HYPERPLASIA (benign prostate hyperplasia): see benign prostate hyperplasia

PSORIASIS: is well known as a cosmetically disfiguring dermatitis (i.e., "the heartbreak of psoriasis"). Psoriasis is characterized by dry, well demarcated silvery, scaling plaques of all sizes that appear primarily behind joints (i.e., elbows and knees) and on the scalp and behind the ears. Celiac disease type changes in the intestines lead to malabsorption of essential nutrients; do a pulse test to determine specific food allergens. Treatment of psoriasis should include avoidance of offending food allergens, rotation diets, folic acid at 15-25 mg per day, vitamin A at 300,000 IU per day as beta carotene, lecithin at 2,500 mg t.i.d. with meals, flaxseed oil at one tbsp. b.i.d., vitamin E at 800-1,200 IU per day, zinc at 50 mg t.i.d., copper at 2 mg per day, selenium at 500-1,000 mcg per day and betaine HCl and pancreatic enzymes at 75-200 mg per day. Topical herbal washes are of palliative value as is topical vitamin A & D creams.

PYORRHEA (periodontal disease): see periodontal disease

Q FEVER: is an acute rickettsial disease caused by Coxiella burnetii and characterized by sudden onset, fever, headache, weakness and pneumonitis. Q fever has a worldwide distribution and is maintained as an endemic infection in domestic animals. Sheep, goats and cattle are the primary reservoirs for human infections. The infection is spread to humans by bites from the infected tick, Dermacentor andersoni and from consuming infected raw milk. Diagnosis is made from a positive blood test. Treatment of Q fever should include tetracycline orally at 250 mg q 4 h (Chloramphenicol may be used in small children to prevent discoloration of permanent teeth by tetracycline).

QUINSY (peritonsillar abscess): is an infection of the tonsil between the tonsil and the pharyngeal constrictor muscle. These infections are rare in children but common in young adults. The "orthodox" EENT will want to do a tonsillectomy — DON'T LET HIM DO IT!!! SAVE YOUR TONSILS!!! Treatment should include vitamin A at 300,000 IU per day as beta carotene, zinc at 50 mg t.i.d., vitamin C to bowel tolerance, gargles with herbal washes, penicillin G or V at 250 mg q 6 h for 12-14 days.

RABBIT FEVER (tularemia): is caused by the bacteria, Francisella tularensis. This disease is contracted by skinning and dressing infected rabbits or ground squirrels (87%); the disease initially appears as a local ulceration at the infection site; the disease secondarily goes systemic causing a typhoid like disease with diarrhea and pneumonia. High fever and recurring chills with drenching sweat are characteristic (I have had tularemia and my grandfather died from it as a result of skinning infected wild rabbits). Diagnosis comes following a high level of suspicion (appropriate history of wild rabbit contact) and the ulcerated primary ulcer at the infection site are enough to make the diagnosis. Sputum cultures are highly infectious and labs should be warned of your suspicions. Treatment of tularemia is with streptomycin IM at 500 mg q 12 h until temperature drops into the normal range; then give tetracycline orally at 250 mg q.i.d. for 10-12 days.

RABIES (hydrophobia): is a highly dangerous viral disease that is transmitted by the blood, tissue (transplanted corneas, livers, kidneys or hearts), urine or saliva of infected animals or people. We are all aware of the dangers of bites from rabies infected bats, foxes, skunks and unvaccinated dogs but most of us are not aware that many cases of fatal rabies occurs following tissue transplants. Rabies in humans is a progressive paralytic disease that is often misdiagnosed as stroke which is why rabies infected tissues get transplanted. Many Americans spend over a hundred dollars to visit the "orthodox" doctor when their child gets bitten by the pet hamster because of fears of rabies — think about it, the incubation period of rabies is fourteen days — if you have had the hamster for three weeks or more rabies is an impossible diagnosis (a free phone call to your veterinarian would be informational and save you a lot of money). High risk research personnel can get preventative vaccinations for rabies. Treatment of rabies should be instituted quickly if success can be anticipated; treatment includes the well known "rabies shots" every day for ten days and respiratory support in a hospital setting.

RACHITIC ROSARY (rickets): is the "beading" of the junction between the ribs and the rib cartilage. This is exclusively a malady of small children who are kept indoors and are not getting an oral source of vitamin D. The rachitic "rosary" is easily palpated. Treatment of the rachitic "rosary" should include oral vitamin D at 400-1,000 IU per day and the base line nutritional supplement program including calcium and magnesium. After the abnormal bony changes become normal, the vitamin D dose should be dropped to 250-400 IU per day; afford daily exposure to sun for at least 30 minutes.

RADIAL NERVE PALSY ("Saturday night palsy"): is the result of compressing the radial nerve against the humerus (this is usually caused by draping the arm over the back of a hard-backed chair for an extended period — i.e., drunken stupor or deep sleep). Radial nerve palsy is characterized by a wrist "drop" and weakness in the ability to extend the wrist and fingers; sometimes there is a loss of sensory function between the first and second fingers. Treatment of radial palsy should include B-complex 50 t.i.d., topical DMSO, acupuncture and hydrotherapy.

RAPE (date rape): is considered by experts to be an act of aggression rather than sexual, however, "date rape" is the result of pent up sexual demands made on a relatively helpless "friend." "Date rape" can be prevented by not going out on couples only dates until the "date" is well known. Group movies, pizza parties and bunking parties are very safe. Go in groups of two or more couples and have the girls dropped off first to the same house or apartment (even better to one of their parents' houses). Prevention of rape requires some extreme action if you are to be effective: 1) knee violently to testicles; 2) mace to the eyes, nose and mouth; 3) keys violently in the eyes; 4) seriously learn martial arts — the "military" bearing acquired sends subliminal messages to leave you alone; 5) get a trained attack dog for jogging, walking and at home; a vicious dog bite to the testicles is a real damper to a rapist; 6) arrange for an apartment "sitter" to be there when you return home; 7) personal weapon that you are prepared to use — this requires practice, practice and more practice and the mind set that you will kill an attacker — pick a small caliber handgun that you are not afraid of and empty the weapon into an attacker; this will prevent him from grabbing it from you and using it against you!!! Carry your weapon with you at all times — "praise the Lord and pass the ammunition!!!" "Treatment" for rape should include an IM injection of dimethyl stilbestrol to initiate a menstrual cycle thus preventing an unwanted pregnancy; counseling may be necessary for women psychologically brutalized; support of friends and lots of positive activity are the best emotional therapy.

RAYNAUD'S DISEASE: is characterized by tingling and numbness in the fingers (and sometimes the nose and tongue) which is caused by spasms of small arteries. The "orthodox" approach to Raynaud's disease is to cut sympathetic nerves and give anesthetics and tranquilizers. Food allergies can be the precipitating factor in Raynaud's disease when arteries are the target tissue; do a pulse test to determine if food allergens are a problem. Rule out "thoracic inlet syndrome" (nerves or arteries coming out of the thorax are squeezed by muscles or bones). Treatment of Raynaud's disease should include calcium and magnesium at 2,000 mg per day and 1,000 mg per day, avoid offending food allergens, avoid caffeine (i.e., coffee, tea, soft drinks, chocolate, etc.), vitamin E at 800-1,200 IU per day, essential fatty acids at 5 gm t.i.d., 1-tryptophane at 500 mg t.i.d., acupuncture, chiropractic and herbs to increase circulation such as cayenne pepper (Capsicum minimum).

RECTAL ITCHING: can be caused by Candidiasis, food allergies, hemorrhoids, crabs, fleas and pinworms. Do a pulse test to rule in or rule out food allergies, take the self test, blood test or skin test to determine Candidiasis. The diagnosis of pinworms requires the Scotch tape test to identify the parasite eggs. The presence of fleas and/or hemorrhoids will require the use of a mirror for self examination of the anal folds. Treatment of rectal itching can be palliated with a variety of herbal washes (see hemorrhoids), Preparation H, sitz baths with herbal washes and/or hydrogen peroxide, specific treatments for parasites.

REYE'S SYNDROME: occurs most frequently in young teens and usually in the fall and winter. Reye's syndrome is characterized by pneumonitis, nausea and vomiting, sudden change in mental status to deep depression, amnesia, agitation to coma and convulsions, fixed dilated pupils and death in 42-80%. The cause of Reye's syndrome is thought to be caused by consumption of aflatoxin (an exotoxin of the grain mold Aspergillus flavus). A typical liver necrosis is present on biopsy; survivors show a 100% recovery of the liver tissue in twelve weeks after the attack. Treatment of Reye's syndrome include barbiturate anesthesia to lower intracranial pressure, IV fluids and electrolytes, pulmonary support, exchange transfusions and dialysis. Vitamin C IV at 5-10 gms per day, B-complex and B-12 IV or IM, selenium IM or IV at 250-500 mcg per day.

RHEUMATIC FEVER: is caused by Streptococcus Group A infection (usually starts as a "strep throat"). Rheumatic fever is characterized by arthritis, skin rash, fever, heart valve inflammation and brain signs (chorea). The residual valve damage is the most dangerous aspect of untreated rheumatic fever. Diagnosis of rheumatic fever is made from the typical symptoms and concurrent positive cultures of Streptococcus Group A. Treatment of rheumatic fever early in the course of the disease will prevent the heart damage. Treatment should include aspirin for joint pain and sulfadiazine orally at 500-1,000 mg/day for 1-2 years or penicillin G or V orally at 250,000 u. b.i.d. for two years.

RHEUMATISM (rheumatoid arthritis): is thought by "orthodox" rheumatologist to be a disease of the immune system; in reality, rheumatoid arthritis is caused initially by an infection by a PPLO (pleuro-pneumonia like organism) or Mycoplasma that characteristically causes an upper respiratory infection and pneumonitis. These organisms secondarily attack the joint membranes of the fingers and toes and later, the larger joints of the shoulders and knees. This disease has been recognized and eliminated in the veterinary industry – again the human population has been left out because the truth would eliminate an entire medical specialty (remember the quote by the famous Dr. Arthur F. Coca — "I am a realist, as long as the profit is in the treatment of symptoms rather than in the search for causes; that's where the medical profession will go for it's harvest.").

Diagnosis of rheumatoid arthritis is made biopsy of the joint membrane, x ray, blood test (elevated SED RATE, positive for RF), and physical examination. The "orthodox" treatment is totally aimed at relieving symptoms (i.e., aspirin, gold shots, steroids); they claim great victory but statistics show that 75% of the rheumatoid arthritis patients improve in the first year without any treatment at all (up to 10% are disfigured and disabled despite "heroic" "orthodox" therapy).

Treatment of rheumatoid arthritis should include specific treatment for Mycoplasma (PPLO) (Minocycline, tetracycline), for six months to one year, IV and/or oral hydrogen peroxide, chelation, acupuncture, enterically coated bromeliad at 40 mg q.i.d., autoimmune urine therapy, DMSO, 1-histidine at 1,000 mg t.i.d., essential fatty acids at 5 gm t.i.d., calcium and magnesium at 2,000 mg and 1,000 mg per day, selenium at 500-1,000 mcg per day, copper at 2-4 mg per day, B-6 at 100 mg t.i.d., catilage at 5 gm t.i.d., acupuncture, hydrotherapy and herbs to include topical camphor (Cinnamonum camphora), black mustard (Brassica nigra), dandelion (Taraxacum officinale), grappie (Harpagophytum procumbens), juniper (Juniperus communis), stinging nettle (Urtica dioica) and sweat vernal grass (Anthoxanthum odoratum). Plant derived colloidal minerals have proved great benefit here.

RICKETS: is caused by a deficiency of vitamin D and is characterized by stunted growth, joint pain and deformed long bones (i.e., bow legs, dropped wristed, "sickle shins," barrel chest, rachitic rosary, etc.).
Treatment of rickets includes supplementation with vitamin D at 400 IU orally, calcium and magnesium at 2,000 mg and 1,000 mg per day, and exposure to sunshine for 30 minutes per day. Advanced cases will require orthotic correction and, in some cases, orthopedic surgery.

RINGING IN THE EARS (Miniars disease, Wallach's vertigo): can be caused by high blood pressure, drug side effects and osteoporosis (fibrous connective tissue squeezing the 8th cranial nerve).
The bones of the body try to get stronger following the loss of mineral by generating connective tissue. The 8th cranial nerve can be squeezed as it passes through the skull into the inner ear. When the vestibular branch is squeezed, vertigo can be a feature; when the auditory branch is squeezed ringing in the ears occurs.
Treatment is directed toward lowering blood pressure, eliminating drug side effects and reversing the osteoporosis with calcium 2000 mg and magnesium 1000 mg, plant derived colloidal trace minerals and 8 to 12 gr of gelatin per day.

RINGWORM: is caused by fungi that invades the skin,

nails and hair; the skin lesions tend to be circular thus the name "ringworm." The organisms most frequently isolated are Micro-sporum (Tinea capitis), Trichophyton (Tinea cruris or jock itch). Cats, rabbits and children are the most common source of infection. Diagnosis is made by seeing the characteristic lesions, culture of the fungi and positive to Woods lamp (lesions of Microsporum will fluoresce a bright pastel green).

Treatment of ringworm should include Griseofulvin orally at 250 mg q.i.d. for four months, vitamin A at 25,000-300,000 IU/day as beta carotene, zinc at 50 mg t.i.d., vitamin E at 800-1,200 IU/day, ultra violet light directly to lesion for up to six minutes per day, and herbs topically including plantain (Plantgo major) and castor oil (Ricinus communis).

ROCKY MOUNTAIN SPOTTED FEVER (tick fever): is caused by a rickettsia (Rickettsia rickettsii) which is transmitted to man by the bite of an infected tick (i.e., the wood tick, Dermacentor andersoni, the dog tick, Dermacentor variabilis, and the lone-star tick, Amblyomma americanum). Rocky Mountain Spotted Fever occurs May through October during the tick season and affects small children who have access to heavily wooded areas directly or indirectly via the family dog who brings home the infected ticks; 90% of the reported cases occur along the Eastern seaboard and only 10% occur in adult hunters from the mountain areas. The symptoms of RMSF follow 7-12 days after a tick bite and are characterized by headaches, chills, weakness, muscle pain, fever, dry cough, skin rash on wrists, ankles, palms, soles and forearms at first then spreads to the neck, face, axilla, buttocks and trunk; liver enlargement and pneumonitis with terminal circulatory failure in untreated cases. DO NOT WAIT FOR A POSITIVE BLOOD

TEST BEFORE INSTITUTING TREATMENT AS DEATH MAY OCCUR AS QUICKLY AS 4-10 DAYS AFTER APPEARANCE OF SYMPTOMS.
Treatment of RMSF should include tetracycline at 500 mg q.i.d. orally or IV if the patient can't swallow capsules. Supportive treatment with IV fluids and electrolytes is essential to rapid and full recovery.

ROSEOLA: is an acute viral disease of infants and toddlers and is characterized by high fever (up to 105 F) and a rash that predominates on the belly and chest and lightly on the face and limbs. Convulsions may occur during the high fever periods. After 3-4 days, the child will feel completely well even though the rash persists. The course of the disease and distribution of the rash are diagnostic.
Treatment of roseola is directed to reducing the fever sufficiently to prevent convulsions and topical poultices on the rash (see measles).

SCABIES (itch): is caused by an almost microscopic "mite" (Sarcoptes scabiei) that burrows into the skin. This mite is very contagious from person to person. The original infestation usually comes from an infected animal or contaminated animal bedding.
Treatment of scabies includes total body application of 1% gamma benzene hexachloride, 25% benzyl benzoate cream in adults and 5-10% sulfur ointment in infants to avoid potential neurotoxicity; poke (Phytolacca decandra) may be used topically as a natural alternative.

SCARLATINA (scarlet fever): is caused by a Streptococcus Group A throat infection. The organism releases a toxin that produces a rash that is most common on the belly, sides and skin folds and a red pulpy "strawberry"

tongue. Fever in the early stages is common; before the advent of antibiotics, deadly epidemics of scarlatina swept through the young populations. Aggressive treatment is recommended to prevent death or rheumatic fever from developing. Diagnosis is made from the characteristic lesions and positive throat cultures of Streptococcus Group A.
Treatment of scarlatina is oral penicillin V at 250 mg q.i.d. for 10-14 days.

SCHIZOPHRENIA ("split" personality): see bi-polar brain disease.

SCIATICA (low back pain radiating down buttocks and legs): can be caused by "subluxations" of lumbar vertebrae, thinning of lumbar inter-vertebral disc, thick wallet in one back pocket; in its most severe form sciatica may be the result of a ruptured intervertebral disc.
Treatment of sciatica should include hydrotherapy, chiropractic, acupuncture, inversion-gravity therapy, calcium and magnesium at 2,000 mg per day and 1,000 mg per day and the baseline nutritional supplement program to include plant derived colloidal minerals .

SCOLIOSIS (curvature of the spine): occurs in preteens and teens (80% in girls) during the rapid growth stages. The patient should be examined bending over facing away from the examiner; the spine is viewed for lateral deviations. Scoliosis may be a benign disease or herald the early stages of muscular dystrophy (MD). Scoliosis is basically caused by one set of the spinal muscles being stronger than the other (i.e., right side stronger than the left) which causes an "S" curve in the spine; these changes are the result of muscle degeneration. Prevention of scoliosis comes with religious consumption of the base line nutritional supplement program. Celiac disease type intestinal damage may be the cause of malabsorption syndromes leading to scoliosis.

Treatment of scoliosis in the early stages will result in a complete cure; failure to aggressively take supplements will result in persistent damage requiring back braces and surgery. Treatment should include avoidance of offending food allergens, vitamin E at 800-1,200 IU per day, selenium at 500-1,000 mcg per day, calcium and magnesium at 2,000 mg and 1,000 mg per day and the base line supplement program to include plant derived colloidal minerals. Chiropractic can be very useful in relieving back muscle spasms associated with scoliosis.

SCURVY (bleeding gums): is caused by a vitamin C deficiency: scurvy may occur concurrently with gingivitis (see periodontitis).

Treatment of scurvy should include vitamin C to bowel tolerance, increase green leafy vegetables and fruit intake, and herbs including dog rose (Rosa canina).

SEBACEOUS CYST (Wen, steatoma): are slow growing benign cystic cutaneous "tumors;" they contain sebaceous material and are frequently found on the scalp (Wen), ears, back or scrotum. The cyst ranges in size from a pea to a golf ball, is firm (like a soft shell egg) and painless.

Treatment of a sebaceous cyst includes a "stab" incision at the lowest edge of the cyst; evacuate the contents; flush with hydrogen peroxide. Large cysts require removal of the cyst wall to prevent refilling of the cyst; place a sterile gauze drain in the empty cyst and gradually remove over a period of 7-10 days.

SEBORRHEIC DERMATIS (dandruff): is a scaling

dermatitis of the scalp and face; the composition and amount of sebum are normal. Celiac disease type intestinal lesions can be the cause of a malabsorption syndrome.

Treatment of seborrheic dermatitis should include biotin at 100 mcg t.i.d., folic acid at 15-25 mg per day, B-6 at 100 mg t.i.d., vitamin E at 800-1,200 mg IU per day, essential fatty acids at 5 gm t.i.d., vitamin A at 300,000 IU per day as beta carotene, zinc at 50 mg t.i.d. and Selson Blue shampoo topically.

SENILE DEMENTIA (senility): see memory loss

SEXUALLY TRANSMITTED DISEASES: include gonorrhea, syphilis, AIDS, Herpes II, warts, etc. SEE EACH DISEASE INDIVIDUALLY. Use condoms, select sexual partners with great care — a mistake can cost you your life!!!

SHARK SKIN (keratosis): is caused by a deficiency of vitamin A and zinc (usually as a result of low animal protein diets). Shark skin is characterized by cracks in the corners of the mouth (cheilosis), oral lesions that are often secondarily infected by Candida albicans (perleche), "geographic" tongue and skin lesions characterized by hard granular plugs resulting from collections of sebaceous and keratinized material in hair follicles which gives a sandpaper — like surface (shark skin).

Treatment of shark skin and related skin problems should include B-complex at 50 mg t.i.d. and skin washes for dermatitis (see dermatitis), vitamin A at 300,000 IU per day as beta carotene, zinc at 50 mg t.i.d. and essential fatty acids at 5 gm t.i.d.

SHINGLES (Herpes zoster): is a chronic viral infection

with the chicken pox virus. The symptoms include a very painful skin lesion ("shingles").
Treatment of shingles should include Isoprinosin at 500-1,500 mg per day and Dermese at 1 q.i.d. and American sarsaparilla (Aralia nudicaulis) as a wash or poultice.

SKIN AILMENTS (dermatitis): are caused by a variety of diseases (see dermatitis).
Treatment of skin disease should include specific treatment for the underlying problem, homeopathy, essential fatty acids at 5 gm t.i.d., vitamin A at 300,000 IU per day as beta carotene, zinc at 50 gm t.i.d., essential fatty acids at 5 gm t.i.d., and herbs including horsetail (Equisetum arvense), pansy (Viola tricolor), Quack grass (Agropyron repens), soap wort (Saponaria officinalis), stinging nettle (Urtica dioica), slippery elm (Ulmus fulva) and globe mallow (Sphaeralcea spp.).

SORE THROAT: can be caused by a variety of viral and bacterial diseases; bacterial diseases (i.e., Streptococcus Group A) tend to exhibit a higher fever than sore throats caused by viral disease (i.e., URI, cold viruses, flu, etc.).
Treatment of sore throats should include antibiotics as necessary for chronic Strep throat and herbs including flax (Linum usitatissimum), garden sage (Salvia officinalis), German chamomile (Matricaria chamomilla), marjoram (Origanum vulgare), marsh-mallow (Althaea officinalis), rosemary (Rosmarinus officinalis), eucalyptus (Eucalyptus globulus), myrtle (Myrica cerifera) and lobelia (Lobelia inflata).

SPRAIN: is characterized by a painful stretching of ligaments of the joints; these traumas can be temporarily debilitating and locally painful. Sprains are caused by lifting, sudden stops or turns and/or trauma.

Treatment of sprains include ice to reduce swelling as immediate first aid, wrap with an Ace bandage for support; fingers may be taped to the adjoining fingers for added support; take cartilage at 5 gm t.i.d., betaine HCl and pancreatic enzymes at 75-200 mg t.i.d. in between meals; DMSO topically, pain gels topically, and herbs including arnica (Arnica montana) and comfrey (Symphytum officinale).

SPIDER BITE: produces swelling, local fever and itching; brown recluse spider bites produce ulceration and require surgical removal.
Treatment for spider bites should include soaking bite wound in a bath prepared from 8-10 sunflowers (Helianthus annus) soaked for 30 minutes.

STRAINS: are more severe than sprains and are characterized by torn ligaments and torn joint capsule with bleeding and swelling. A very painful joint trauma; emergency treatment should include ice to reduce swelling; strains frequently require a cast similar to that used for a fracture to immobilize and rest the injured joint.
Treatment of strains should include ice, DMSO, pain gels, betaine HCl and pancreatic enzymes at 75-200 mg t.i.d. between meals and herbs including arnica (Arnica montana), comfrey (Symphytum officinale) and lavender (Lavandula spp.). A cast and crutches are appropriate to provide support and rest.

STOMACH DISORDERS: see dyspepsia

STRESS: is the body's reaction to stressors (i.e., overwork, money problems, marriage problems, etc.). The adrenals in particular suffer from stress resulting in a lowering of the immune systems ability to protect you

from infection, cancer, and disturbs the function of your entire endocrine system including energy management (i.e., blood sugar, blood pressure, thyroid, etc.).
Treatment of stress should include relaxation, subliminal distress audio tapes, sublingual ACE drops at 5-10 drops t.i.d., vitamin C to bowel tolerance, zinc at 50 mg t.i.d., learn to compartmentalize time expenditure, have 20 projects (a combination of work, family and hobbies — remember the old saying "about giving the project to the busiest person if you want it done."

STROKE (cerebrovascular accident, CVA): is the result of a blood clot or tumor blocking an artery supplying the brain. The result is local brain tissue death from the lack of oxygen and food. If the damaged area is small enough and not in a vital area the brain will reroute the brain's functions to unused portions through a relearning and compensation process.
Treatment of stroke should include EDTA chelation and IV hydrogen peroxide as soon as possible, essential fatty acids at 5 gm t.i.d., exercise and the base line nutritional supplement program to include plant derived colloidal minerals.

SWEAT TEST: a nonspecific test that measures the amount of electrolytes (i.e., sodium, chlorides and potassium) in sweat; originally it was to be a specific genetic test for cystic fibrosis (CF); however, today it has been found to be positive in 17 different diseases, food allergies, starvation, kwashiorkor, celiac disease, etc. The mechanism is related to essential fatty acid deficiencies and thus the lack of certain prostaglandins (short lived hormone — like substances) which control sweat electrolyte levels.

SWIMMERS EAR: is usually caused by Candida albicans growing in the external ear canal; constant dampness during the summer swimming season is thought to be the underlying cause.
Treatment for swimmers ear include hydrogen peroxide ear drops and/or Nystatin ear drops.

SYPHILIS: is a sexually transmitted disease caused by the spirochete Treponema palli-dum; it has been associated with 90% of AIDS patients in one study of homosexual males. Syphilis is characterized by active infection and by years of spontaneous remission. Symptoms of syphilis include a primary lesion or chancre sore that may persist for 3-4 months on the penis, vulva, lips, tongue, etc.; skin rashes appear after 3-4 months and last for weeks to months; 80% of infected people have herpes-like sores on lips, tongue, penis or vulva; the disease may infect any organ including liver, bone, brain, eyes, heart, etc. Terminal stages of tertiary syphilis occurs 10-25 years after the original infection. Diagnosis is made from a positive blood VDRL test.
Treatment for syphilis is specific in all stages with penicillin G at 2.4 million u IM with a second treatment 10-14 days later. Like AIDS, syphilis is a reportable disease to the Public Health Service.

TACHYCARDIA (rapid heartbeat): is characterized by rapid heartbeat; tachycardia can be caused by "nervous heart," hyperthyroidism, food allergies, hypoglycemia, nutritional deficiencies (i.e., B-1, B-3, selenium, etc.), poisons and organic heart disease. A classic example is allergy to MSG or "Chinese Restaurant Syndrome."
Treatment of tachycardia should include the identification and treatment of the underlying cause (see laboratory and diagnostic section; acupuncture, selenium at

500-1,000 mcg per day, B-1 at 100 mg t.i.d., B-3 at 450 mg t.i.d. as time release tablets, subliminal relaxation tapes and herbs including English hawthorn (Crataegus oxyacantha), hops (Humulus lupulus), lavender (Lavandula angustifolia), mother wort (Leonurus cardiaca), valerian (Valeriana officinalis) and lily-of-the-valley (Convallariana magalis).

TAPEWORMS (cestodes): can set up housekeeping in your intestines without causing any noticeable problem in a well nourished person and can cause wasting weight loss and anemia. Tapeworms are contracted by eating contaminated watercress, raw fish, raw beef or raw pork. The encysted larvae are released into the digestive tract and attach to the intestinal wall by suckers or hooks in their head. Diagnosis of tapeworms may be made by seeing segments on the surface of the bowel movement (look like grains of rice that are moving), or observing eggs in microscopic examination of the stool (see parasites in laboratory section). Prevention of tapeworms is related to cooking fish and meat before consumption and thoroughly washing vegetables.

Treatment of tapeworms requires the use of a single dose of niclosamide at 2 gm taken with a glass of water. Recheck stool in 3-6 months for reinfestation. Retreat if needed. Herbs may be helpful including garlic (Allium sativum) and male fern (Dryopteris Felix-mas); pretreating herbal remedies for tapeworms with a teaspoon of castor oil in the morning before treatment increases the efficiency.

TARDIVE DYSKINESIA (spasms of facial muscles): is on the increase as a side effect of heavy tranquilizer (phenothiazines) usage.

Treatment of tardive dyskinesia should include the

discontinuation of the inducing drugs, B-3 at 450 mg t.i.d. as time release tablets, phosphatidyl choline at 30 gm per day, B-6 at 200 mg q.i.d., essential fatty acids at 5 gm t.i.d., manganese at 10-15 mg per day, vitamin E at 800-1,200 IU per day.

TEETH DISCOLORATION (tetracyclines): with reduced enamel thickness is a common side effect of prolonged administration of tetracyclines during the second half of pregnancy or during early tooth development; the affected teeth will be brown or gray and fluorescent orange-green in ultraviolet light. Prevention is the name of the game; cosmetic capping is necessary if permanent teeth are affected.

TEETHING: can be an uncomfortable event for infant and parents with painful local swellings, sudden fever, irritability and diarrhea (especially irritating with severe diaper rash).

Treatment of teething includes tylenol or aspirin drops (follow label directions) and herbs including German chamomile (Matricaria chamomilla) as teaspoon doses as needed.

TMJ (temporal-mandibular joint syndrome): is characterized by headaches, misalignment of teeth, popping the TM joints while talking or eating, etc. This syndrome is related to carpal tunnel syndrome and repetitive motion syndrome in that all three are caused by deficiencies of arsenic, manganese and choline.

Treat for osteoporosis and be sure to include colloidal arseni and manganese and choline.

TESTICULAR ATROPHY: is not uncommon in aging men or following an episode of mumps. Testicular atrophy may result in decreased sexual drive and feminization.

Treatment of testicular atrophy should include zinc at 50 mg t.i.d., plant derived colloidal minerals, an herbal combination mixed with testosterone (Zumba), ginseng (Panax ginseng) and saw palmetto (Sarenoa serrulata).

THALLIUM POISONING (rat or insect baits): can accidentally occur when small children get into pesticides containing thallium salts. Thallium poisoning can be rapidly fatal if not treated promptly. Symptoms include bloody vomiting and diarrhea, oral irritations with severe salivation, tremors, facial palsy and hair loss in 3-4 weeks in survivors.

Treatment for thallium poisoning should include contact with poison control centers; syrup of ipecac to induce vomiting at 15-30 ml (1-2 tbsp.) for children and adults; follow with several pints of water until vomiting occurs, one tbsp. activated charcoal in a glass of water, control convulsions diazepam. Chelation therapy is of no value for thallium poisoning.

THRUSH (oral candidiasis): is an oral yeast infection caused by Candida albicans; thrush is characterized by creamy white patches that can be scrapped off with a tongue depressor. Candida albicans is an ubiquitous nonpathogenic yeast under normal circumstances which becomes pathogenic and invades tissue when the hosts ability to defend itself is lost (i.e., malnutrition, chemotherapy, AIDS, etc.) or the competing intestinal organisms are killed out (i.e., antibiotic therapy, etc.). Diagnosis can be made from the characteristic lesions or by looking at the exudate under the microscope.

Treatment of thrush includes the use of oral washes and gargling with hydrogen peroxide; small infants unable to gargle may have to have topical Nystatin applied to the lesions. The underlying condition must also be dealt with to allow you to defend yourself against reinfection. Vitamin C to bowel tolerance, selenium at 25-1,000 mcg per day, vitamin E at 800-1,200 IU per day, vitamin A at 25,000-300,000 IU per day as beta carotene and zinc at 50 mg t.i.d. are of great value in restoring the immune status. Following extended antibiotic therapy (i.e., acne, rheumatic fever, cystic fibrosis, etc.) you can restore the competitive organisms into the bowel (to help keep yeast numbers down) by the use of Lactobacillus acidophilus; administer Lactobacillus at ten capsules twice each day between meals for ten days each month to restore normal colon count.

TINNITUS (ringing or buzzing in the ear): is characterized by a ringing or buzzing in the ear. "Orthodox" doctors suggest that "surgery is of no value; if you can't tolerate the ringing, play background music." In reality, there are a variety of causes of tinnitus including hypertension, lead, mercury toxicity, nutritional deficiencies, osteoporosis, food allergies and/or hypoglycemia. Do the necessary laboratory work to make a specific diagnosis including the pulse test, six-hour GTT and hair analysis. Take the base line nutritional program.
Treatment of tinnitus should include the treatment of the underlying disease, avoid offending food allergens, autoimmune urine therapy, avoid sugar and all refined foods, zinc at 50 mg t.i.d., tin from plant derived colloidal minerals, essential fatty acids at 5 gm t.i.d., vitamin A at 300,000 IU per day as beta carotene, calcium and magnesium at 2,000 and 1,000 mg per day and betaine HCl and pancreatic enzymes at 75-200 mg t.i.d. 15 minutes before meals.

TIREDNESS (chronic fatigue syndrome): see chronic fatigue syndrome

TONSILLITIS: is characterized by an inflamed sore throat caused by viruses or Streptococcus organisms.
Treatment of tonsillitis should include hydrogen peroxide mouthwash and gargle, vitamin C to bowel tolerance, vitamin C at 25,000-300,000 IU per day as beta carotene, zinc at 50 mg t.i.d., selenium at 25-1,000 mcg per day, herbs to include green hellebore (Veratrum viride), marshmallow (Althaea officinalis), flaxseed (Linum usitatissimum), German chamomile (Matricaria chamomilla), marjoram (Origanum vulgare) garden sage (Salvia officinalis).

TOOTHACHE: is usually caused by cavities (caries) that are stimulated to pain by sweets, cold or hot drinks.
Treatment of caries and toothache should include filling of the tooth with enamel amalgams, avoid stimuli that initiates pain, acupuncture and herbs to include penny royal (Mentha pulegium), lavender (Lavandula spp.), gelsemium (Gelsemium nitidum), as necessary OTC analgesics (i.e., aspirin, tylenol, tylenol-3).

TORTICOLLIS SPASMODIC (wryneck): is caused by spasms of the neck muscles and/or "subluxations" of the cervical vertebrae. Torticollis may be caused by "whiplash" injuries, calcium deficiencies and/or muscular dystrophy.
Treatment of torticollis should include chiropractic, massage therapy, hydro-therapy, acupuncture, calcium and magnesium at 2,000 and 1,000 mg per day, selenium at 500-1,000 mcg per day and vitamin E at 800-1,200 IU per day.

TOXIC SHOCK SYNDROME (TSS): is caused by an exotoxin produced by a Staphylococcus organism; the exotoxin is similar if not identical to that which is produced by Staph food poisoning. Approximately 15% of those affected are men; the remainder are young women between 13-32 years of age. The syndrome is precipitated by improper use of vaginal tampons (use of a single tampon for longer than four hours produces an ideal environment for Staphylococcus growth. TSS is characterized by high fever, sudden onset, vomiting, diarrhea, confusion, skin rash, headache, sore throat with rapid deterioration and death within 48 hours. Prevention is the best policy with TSS; avoid prolonged use of individual tampons and avoid food poisoning by proper food handling.

Treatment of toxic shock syndrome is a medical emergency requiring rapid emergency room care — DO NOT LET THEM MAKE YOU WAIT IN THE HALL. Treatment should include IV fluids and electrolytes, as well as penicillin to kill the Staphylococcus.

TOXOPLASMOSIS (cat coccidia): is caused by an intermediate stage of a house cat intestinal protozoa (Isospora bigemina); the intermediate stage in humans was originally named Toxoplasma gondii and the "orthodox" doctors refuse to admit that it is a cat parasite. "Toxoplasmosis" in man is characterized by a generalized and/or a brain disease; toxoplasmosis is acquired in man from inhaling or swallowing dust from contaminated "kitty litter" boxes or outdoor sand piles or from eating rare beef. "Toxoplasmosis" is of particular danger to pregnant women as infection will cause birth defects in the fetus (i.e., brain defects, blindness, mental retardation); symptoms in adults can mimic the flu, cause headache, rash, high fever, swollen lymph nodes, meningitis, hepatitis, pneumonitis, myocarditis, blindness and diarrhea. Diagnosis of "toxoplasmosis" is made from a positive blood test or skin test following a high level of suspicion. Prevention of "toxoplasmosis" in pregnant women is related to avoiding cats just prior to, and during, pregnancy (i.e., move cat to grandma's house temporarily) and eating well-cooked meats.

Treatment of "toxoplasmosis" should include trisulfapyrimidine orally at 25 mg (1 mg/kg for kids) daily for four weeks.

TRIGLYCERIDES (ELEVATED): can be a sign of diabetes as well as liver problems. Do a six-hour GTT and a full blood chemistry. Elevated triglycerides is a high risk factor for cardiovascular disease and stroke. Do a pulse test to determine if food allergies are involved.

Treatment of elevated triglycerides should include moderate exercise (walking), avoidance of sugar, avoidance of refined foods, essential fatty acids at 5 gm t.i.d., high fiber and raw foods diet, eliminate red meat, chromium at 100-200 mcg t.i.d., selenium at 500-1,000 mcg per day, plant derived colloidal minerals, vitamin C to bowel tolerance and the base line nutritional supplement program.

ULCER (stomach): is brought on by an infection with *Helicobactor pylori*. Antibiotics for 4 to 6 weeks are a preferred treatment of gastric ulcers over surgery.

Treatment of gastric ulcers should include alfalfa (Medicago sativa), for its {vitamin U" factor, bioflavonoids at 1,000 mg q.i.d., B-6 at 100 mg t.i.d., vitamin A at 300,000 IU per day as beta carotene, zinc at 20 mg t.i.d., glutamine at 400 mg q.i.d., avoid alcohol, avoid sugar and refined foods, consume a high nutritional fiber diet. Antibiotics are a preferred treatment of gastric ulcers over surgery. At any sign of "coffee grounds" vomiting, get to an emergency room immediately as this is a sign of a hemorrhaging ulcer.

ULCERATIVE COLITIS (Crohn's Disease): see Crohn's Disease

URTICARIA (food allergy rash): see food allergies

VAGINITIS (vaginal discharge): can be caused by a great variety of diseases and syndromes ranging from panty-hose without ventilation, parasites (Trichomonas vaginalis), yeast infections (Candida albicans), venereal disease (gonorrhea, syphilis), etc. Diagnosis of the specific underlying disease is essential to correct therapy. History will be useful as well as vaginal cultures.
Treatment of vaginitis should include specific therapy following diagnostic procedures (see specific diseases). For nonspecific vaginitis you may use hydrogen peroxide douches twice weekly, vinegar douches (two tbsp./ pint of warm water), yogurt douches and herbs to include myrtle (Myrica cerifera) and blue cohosh (Caulophyllum thalictroides).

VARICOSE VEINS: are thought to be caused by constipation and constant vertical posture; copper deficiency may also be a contributing factor.
Treatment of varicose veins should include vitamin C to bowel tolerance, vitamin E at 800-1,200 IU per day, zinc at 50 mg t.i.d., bioflavonoids at 600 mg t.i.d., DMSO, hydrotherapy, copper at 2 mg per day (try a copper bracelet) and herbs including marigold (Calendula officinalis) topically, rue (Ruta graveolens), yellow sweet clover (Uelilotus officinalis).

VERTIGO (dizziness, car sickness, motion sickness):

see Car Sickness, Wallach's Vertigo. Take powdered peppercorns (Piper nigrum).

VITILIGO (loss of skin color): is a loss of skin color, especially in dark or black skinned people.
Treatment of vitiligo should include extracts of placenta, live cell therapy, PABA at 100 mg q.i.d., phenylalanine at 50 mg/kg/day, copper at 2 mg per day, copper bracelet, vitamin A at 300,000 IU pr day as beta carotene, zinc at 50 mg t.i.d., Vitamin B-12 at 2000 mcgs per day, folic acid l mg per day and the base line nutritional supplementation program to include plant derived colloidal minerals.

WALLACH' S VERTIGO (dizziness with or without ringing in the ears): Osteoporosis of the skull. The connective tissue generated by the demineralized bones squeezes the vestibular branch of the 8th cranial nerve.
Treatment approach includes osteoporosis nutritional program — chondroitin sulfate (gelatin), calcium 200 mg, 1000 mg magnesium, Boron one mg and plant derived colloidal minerals containing all 60 essential minerals.

WARTS (papillomas): contagious (viral) benign skin tumors — warts (verrucae vulgaris), planter warts (verrucae on the sole of the foot), venereal warts (condylomata acuminata) may be found on the vulva and penis.
Treatment of warts should include topical application of cashew nut (Anacardium occidentale), oil of yellow cedar (Thuja occidentalis) and milk-weed juice. There are commercial wart removal kits available from your pharmacy that employ salacylic acid topically.

WEIGHT LOSS: see diets

WHITE SPOTS, FINGERNAILS: are caused by zinc deficiency. Treatment should include zinc at 50 mg t.i.d.; take the base line nutritional program to include plant derived colloidal minerals.

WORMS (parasites): see parasites
Treatment may include wormwood (Artemisia absinthium), and butternut (Juglans cinerea). Levamisol is a good veterinary "wormer" that can be used very effectively in humans with minimal to no side effects.

WOUNDS (chronic ulcers): treat topically with herbs including euphorbia (Chamaesyce spp.), cliff rose (Allionia coccinea), arnica (Arnica montana), snake root (Aristolochia clematitis), German chamomile (Matricaria chamomilla), marigold (Calendula officinalis), snake root (Sanicula europaea) and witch hazel (Hamamelis virginiana)

ZITS (pimples, acne): see acne

Chapter 11

Referrals

"An unavoidable conclusion is that the way in which our medical care system has evolved has created conditions that increased the likelihood of damage to the patient."

— Rick Carlson
The End of Medicine

One of your responsibilities as your own "primary health care provider" is to recognize when you need the advice and counsel of a "specialist." An obvious example would be if you were run over by a concrete truck you will need an orthopedic surgeon "to put you back together again." On the other hand, you don't need an EENT if you have an earache three times per year. "Orthodox" doctors love to "specialize" in allergies since their patients rarely have a life threatening allergy (that is the "orthodox" attitude about allergies) and they keep coming back forever for allergy shots and new nasal sprays!"

Specialists in the "orthodox" medical field tend to be a very fickle "kiss and run" bunch who rarely get a direct inquiry from a patient; in fact, in many cases you would be anesthetized or tranquilized in the hospital the first time you get interviewed by "your specialist" (in some cases you meet him after the "procedure" is complete — you couldn't even pick him out of a "line up" if you had to). "Specialist" depend on the "other" "orthodox" doctors to feed them "grist" for the "mill." It's kind of like one car salesman asking another to help you pick out options on a new car!

"Specialists" tend to be the speakers at "continuing education" seminars that "orthodox doctors are forced to go to each year to maintain their license. In this way, the "specialists" keep their name and "wares" in front of their "sales force" (the "snake oil" huckster on the back of the wagon is pitching to the "orthodox" doctors!!!).

"Specialist" should be highly skilled at mechanical procedures since they only do one or two, but beware. Remember the old saying, "those who can — do and those who can't — teach;" well, in "orthodox" medicine it's those who can-do and those who can't-specialize."

"Specialists" rarely "see the forest for the trees;" there are a variety of reasons for this. There is a certain amount of "tunnel vision" in all of us, especially when our livelihood is at stake! If an "orthodox" doctor refers you to a surgeon to have your feet amputated for diabetic ulcers, the surgeon is not going to suggest a hyperbaric oxygen chamber to save your feet — he's a surgeon! The horror of this is he will sleep well and play happily with his girlfriend believing that he did you a service.

A second reason why the "specialist" can't "see the forest for the trees" is as a group they have a problem. It is well documented that "22,600 - 33,600 are alcoholics, recovering alcoholics or soon to be alcoholics." "Alcoholism is a primary disease to which physicians as a group, seem highly susceptible and often goes hand in hand with drug abuse" so says Stephen C. Scheiber, M.D. in *The Impaired Physician.*

A recent Harvard study has revealed that "59% of physicians 78% of medical students use psychoactive drugs (usually marijuana and cocaine) and that 40% of "orthodox" doctors get "high" with friends on a regular basis; lastly, the United States loses the equivalent of seven medical school graduating classes each year to drug addiction, alcoholism and suicide.

In the book, *Medicine On Trial*, they calculate that patients visit these "ticking time bomb" "orthodox" physicians at least 45-100 million times each year!

We like the old country doctor or the veterinary approach; the closer the doctor is to his patient, the less likely it is they will do them harm (it is highly unlikely that you will harm yourself as your own "primary health care provider"). The veterinarian does his own anesthesia, obstetrics, surgery, dentistry, internal medicine, gastroenterology, EENT, pediatrics, cardiology, radiology, etc. (just like "ole Doc Adams" on Gunsmoke). Are veterinarians smarter or more capable than "orthodox" doctors? Probably so!!! We know for sure they love their patients more!

If the "skills" of a "specialist" are required, get three (3) or more opinions from three (3) or more different "specialists" (be sure to ask one from a totally different field as they will be more likely to give you an objective view) as this will increase your chances of survival. After all, you get three bids for a body repair on a car for an insurance company and three bids for a house painting contract, don't you??

The more "exotic" the "specialist," the greater the risk to you; it's like playing poker with $100 bills instead of matches. A surgeon who does laminectomies for low back problems is not going to refer you to a chiropractor for more conservative (and more effective) approaches (especially if his Mercedes payment is due).

Ask the "specialist" to speak to ten of his patients who have gone through the procedure. "Orthodox" doctors don't like this approach, as "testimonials are not scientific;" this may be true but it certainly will give you an idea if ten patients survived the procedure (or if, in fact, he has even done this procedure before!)

Many "specialists" will not accept you for a patient unless you are "referred" by an "orthodox" doctor; however, because the "patient pool" of the 80s is dwindling (educated people can't be sold the Brooklyn Bridge) this is changing — if not yourself, then your chiropractor or naturopathic physician (or even your veterinarian) can refer you.

Beware of "specialists" who brag about doing their procedure on their colleague's pet dog or hamster — if he had enough patients because of exceptional skills, he wouldn't have enough time for such frivolity.

If you have two or more "doctors" in your "family practice" you can "specialize" in diagnostic techniques as well as therapy modalities. My family did; my grandmother took care of the flu, sore throats, croup, etc. and my mother loved to do the "surgery" (remove splinters, etc.). We are lucky in our "family practice;" we have two "specialists" neither of whom smoke, drink or "get high." One of us is interested in internal medicine and nutrition while the other specializes in surgery and Traditional Chinese Medicine. This way we get two sober opinions on each problem and, as a result, we are less often in need of outside "help" and are certainly less likely to get injured.

If you do need an outside doctor, contact your naturopathic physician or chiropractor for advice; start out at the conservative end of the "stick." We get so many patients who have been "cut," "burned" and "poisoned" and have their insurance exhausted by the "orthodox" medical system, then they turn to us for help. The amazing thing is we can help, even at this late stage. Ask about and pursue alternative therapies before you get damaged!

We collect obituaries of MD's as a hobby — not only do they remind us that MD's are mortal but also that they are not very good examples of their trade. MD's die of the strangest things such as heart attacks while jogging in the park, cancer, diabetes, liver cirrhosis and drug over doses (we think this is more fun than collecting stamps or baseball cards!). The real value of this collection is that it continually gives us confidence in advising you to be your own doctor!!!

Be bold! It is time to commit! It is time to become so independent that the "orthodox" doctors will begin to put fliers on windshields of cars in the mall parking lots. Let the free enterprise system that made America great help make our health great! Separate medicine and state!!!

Chapter 12
Insurance & Hospitals

> *"They almost killed me, he thought; and he felt his heart pound with dangerous rage. But there was no J'accuse. At some point, it seemed to him, human failure melted into and became inseparable from institutional failure, the two together forging such a formidable instrument for failure as to dictate more horror stories than the public ever dreamed of."*
>
> – Martha Weinman Lear
> *Heartsounds*

The best insurance is not to get sick! This is not only less time consuming but it is also cheaper than illness (we are sure you already know this by now). The veterinary profession has long ago learned that it was cheaper to put a little calcium in the feed to prevent arthritis than it was to give gold shots to the prize bull. The veterinarians job is to do the best job possible for the animal patient and save the farmer money. We just don't see this effort in "orthodox" hospitals which have become like Star Trek robots running amuck sucking up patients for organ "donors" and then having the gall to bill the "donor's" family $250,000 for extended ICU use. This is like paying the car dealership to steal your car!

An independent survey was done of "orthodox" hospital insurance billing in 1,000 hospitals and it was found that 97% or 970 sent out incorrect insurance billings, the interesting part of the study was that 100% of the "mistakes" were in the favor of the hospital (come on now, what are the odds that this is a computer error — somewhere around 200 billion to one — in other words, they tried to rip off the insurance companies!). This "soiling of the nest" is a sure sign that they are in the process of dying out. It appears that the "orthodox" hospital is a terminal relic of ancient history.

Quackery can be defined as "that which claims too much," says Stephen Benett, M.D. If this is so, then hospitals are full of "quacks!" It is safer at home than at a hospital (everyone will agree to that). As much as 50% of all new equipment in hospitals is defective when it's delivered (i.e., anesthesia machines, fetal cardiac monitors, infusion pumps, etc.) Eighty to 90% of all anesthetic deaths are due to human error (do the anesthesiologists tell you that? Hell, no! If they did, no one would ever submit to a general anesthesia). A minimum of 100,000 deaths from "nosocomial" infections (hospital caused) occur each year and another 100,000 have "nosocomial" blood infections each year but recover because of antibiotics. This has led the summary of one Harvard study to state "doctor induced infection is among the top ten leading causes of death in the United States today!"

The veterinarian with statistics like these would starve to death. No farmer in his right mind would keep calling when he got "service" that didn't benefit his animals or his P & L statement! There are no insurance companies to pay the veterinarian, he must deal directly with the farmer and no TV ads saying what a wonderful guy he is will induce the farmer to call him if he can't deliver a worthwhile service. The same is not true for the "orthodox" doctor; the insurance companies keep on paying and then raise our insurance rates because of the "high cost of medical services;" if you buy a typewriter and it doesn't work, you return it and get a refund. When the insurance company pays, most people don't ask the orthopedic surgeon for a refund if the hip replacement fails because they don't feel that it came out of their own pocket. This then is why veterinarians give better service — they are directly responsible to the purchaser of that service. Are veterinarians smarter than "orthodox" doctors? Probably so! We know for sure that its harder to get into veterinary school than medical school and that veterinarians love their patients more!

Why don't veterinarians have a high rate of "nosocomial" infections; animals are certainly less hygienic than humans. The reason is simple; they expect a certain amount of contamination and compensate for it by giving "preventive" doses of antibiotics during surgery. This eliminates the infections!!! The reason "orthodox" doctors don't do this is simply arrogance. They wash their hands 5-10 minutes (but they wear their scrubs to the hospital cafeteria) and they feel that all should be well if they wear sterile gloves. It would be interesting to use the veterinary technique of "preventative" antibiotics with surgery in ten hospitals and compare their "nosocomial" infection rate with ten hospitals that don't (a fourth grade biologist can figure out the answer to this one even before the experiment — "It's elementary, Watson!!!").

"Health Insurance" should be called "Sickness Insurance" because they only pay out when you are sick; even boat or auto insurance lowers your rates or gives you a year end rebate if you don't use the insurance! If you want the lowest rates of health insurance today you should join the Christian Science Church; they don't consume alcohol, smoke, they have a great diet and exercise program and they avoid prescription drugs, blood transfusions, etc.!!!

If you want insurance coverage for "alternative" health care (i.e., naturopathic physicians, chiropractic physicians, homeopathic physicians and alternative treatment modalities) you can find it; however, it will be added onto your "basic health" plan as a very expensive "rider." The "rider" usually costs more than the "basic plan." This high cost is not because "alternative care" costs more (on the contrary — it always costs less!!) but rather the insurance companies have a "sweetheart deal" with the "orthodox" doctors under the guise of "we want to protect you from quacks." Additionally, insurance companies pay for services only approved by their medical committees which are dominated by MD's — put some ND's or DC's on the insurance committee and see what gets paid for!!!

True "preventative medicine" through healthful living, base line nutritional supplement programs (to include plant derived colloidal minerals) and constant self-care is the best insurance buy for your health dollars.

The good news is there is a movement afoot today to start health cooperatives that offer alternative health care that have accident riders added to them. In our opinion, this is long over due and is sure to be an instant hit.

If you have to be in the hospital, insist on having a spouse, parent or child stay with you to check out each shot, each pill and each procedure before it is administered to you. Also, they can make sure that you don't get "dropped through the cracks" and left out in the hall for hours after having an x ray, surgery or therapy. They can make sure you are eating properly, that your IVs are hooked up properly, get blood from your own family if needed. This may sound extreme to you but since "orthodox" doctors do this for their families, they must know something they aren't telling us!!! The reason why "doctors make the worst patients" is they know what is and what isn't happening in hospitals and they don't want to be just another statistical victim!!!

Chapter 13
Public Health

> *"Thoughtful public discussion of the iatrogenic pandemic, beginning with an insistence upon demystification of all medical matters, will not be dangerous to the common health. Indeed, what is dangerous is a passive public that has come to rely on superficial medical house cleaning."*
>
> — Ian Illich

The government can no longer ensure the public health, either from the environmental disaster or the "orthodox" Bermuda Triangle (FDA, AMA and drug companies). For the last five years, the "medical industrial" Bermuda Triangle has cost the American people more than the Pentagon and national defense budget! Yet, Americans are rated 17th in longevity, 19th in healthfulness, 23rd in live births and first year survivability and 32nd in birth defects when compared with the western industrialized nations by the WHO. The 20 countries that are healthier than us have a total gross national product of less than what we spend for medical care. "It is elementary, Watson;" we are not getting equitable value for our health care dollar!!! We have changed the American economic systems from "guns and butter" to "guns and pharmaceuticals!!!" It is of interest that the government agency that came forward in 1992 and said that all sexually active women should be taking vitamins and minerals before conception to prevent birth defects was the CDC (Center for Disease Control) — not the FDA ! It makes sense though — the CDC is beholding to no one or no company for generating revenues as is the FDA!

When AT&T had a monopoly on the long distance fees and telephone equipment rentals, the rates sky-rocketed (it's the nature of the beast to charge whatever the market will bear). The government finally deregulated them and actually split them up into smaller regional companies and encouraged new competitive companies to emerge and let the market place decide the costs and services needed. Within two years, the quality of service improved and AT&T dropped their costs to meet those of the competition. It is amazing what true free enterprise does for the consumer. We are convinced that the best interest of the American people would be preserved if there is a separation of "Medicine" and "State" just like there is a separation of "Church" and "State!!!"

The monopoly must end. No surgery without rebates ("no taxation without representation"). Don't operate on me ("Don't Tread on Me"). Give me alternative health care or give me death ("Give me liberty or give me death"). These homey little sayings are what triggered the "Boston Tea Party;" isn't it time for a "Boston (herbal) tea party?"

The environment is another public health concern from the micro environment of our homes (i.e., contaminated food, contaminated water, chlorine, formaldehyde, Radon gas, chlorinated hydrocarbons, etc.) to the national environment burdened with industrial and medical wastes. We have established rules and regulations to ensure laboratory animals health and well-being down to the air flow exchanges per hour, water and food quality, numbers per square foot, lightening quality, etc.; doesn't it seem odd that we can solve all of these problems for laboratory animals and not for ourselves.

As unlikely as it sounds, the Bermuda Triangle (FDA, AMA and drug companies) have threads in common with the solving of the environmental crisis. In each case, we must take matters into our own hands! Not only must we become our own "primary health care provider" but we must also take on the responsibility for our own household "micro" environment! This means dropping our personal pollution load to a minimum by growing a certain amount of our own "organic" food, we must have home water treatment systems and air conditioning systems in the fullest sense (not just cooling), energy conservation (i.e., home solar power, wind power generation for the home where appropriate).

Home water treatment systems are no longer an elective luxury; they have, in fact, become necessary to life itself. There are more than 3,000 chemicals in our drinking and bathing water that are not removed by present community water treatment systems (just because the water is clear doesn't mean that it is safe!). Almost all of these chemicals are carcinogenic. The types of filters required to remove all of these chemicals are too slow for the volume of water required by general use. We must do it ourselves or become a cancer statistic twice (first for getting cancer from our drinking water and second killed by the "cut," "burn" and "poison" surgery, radiation and chemotherapy of "orthodox" medicine!!!); these carcinogens are insidious, they are colorless and odorless but deadly! A filter with bone charcoal will remove all of the hydrocarbons and heavy metals.

Air treatment is another essential system in your home. Remember, you spend a minimum of eight hours or 33 1/3% of your day in the home (housewives spend as much as 90% of their day in the house! Women also have an overall higher cancer rate than men! "It's elementary, Watson").

In Europe and Asia, it is common for city dwellers to raise a portion of their own food; not only is it a healthful, relaxing hobby but it is also an economical hobby. It guarantees you a portion of your food intake is organically grown thus reducing your pollution intake from food sources. Vegetables are easy for the beginner including carrots, bell peppers, radishes, tomatoes, lettuce, cabbage, etc.; meats can include rabbits, pigeons, chickens, eggs, fish, etc. At retirement, this "hobby" will turn into a big dividend on your fixed income and you can sell your "surplus!!!"

Be sure to include plant derived colloidal minerals into your public health program — they prevent disease and reduce your risk of damage from heavy metals and pollution in the environment!

Don't wait for a "Love Canal" incident in your community before you get concerned. Remember, "This Is Your Life!" Be bold, take control of your own destiny, your own health and your own household's "Public Health."

References & Resources

Blackie, Margery. *The Patient, Not the Cure. The Challenge of Homeopathy.* Woodbridge Press Publishing Company, Santa Barbara, California. 1977

Carter, Mildred. *Hand Reflexology: The Key to Perfect Health.* Parker Publishing Company, Inc. West Nyack, New York. 1981

Coca, Arthur. *The Pulse Test: The Secret of Building Your Basic Health.* Lyle Stuart, Inc. Secaucus, N.J. 1982

Ferm, Max and Ferm, Betty. *How to Save Your Dollars With Generic Drugs.* William Marrow and Company, Inc. New York. 1985

Fredericks, Carlton and Goodman, Herman. *Low Blood Sugar and You.* Constellation International, 51 Madison Avenue, New York, N.Y. 1969

Heinerman, John. *Science of Herbal Medicine.* BiWorld Publishing Company. 1979

Inlander, Charles, Levin, Lowell and Weiner, Ed. *Medicine on Trial*. Prentice Hall Press, New York. London. Toronto. 1988

Leek, Sybil. *Herbs: Medicine and Mysticism.* Henry Regnery Company, Chicago. 1975

Mendelsohn, Robert. *Male Practice: How Doctors Manipulate Women*. Contemporary Books, Inc., Chicago. 1981

Pelton, Ross. *Mind Food and Smart Pills.* T & R Publishers, Poway, California. 1986

Stoff, Jesse and Pellegrino, Charles. *Chronic Fatigue Syndrome: The Hidden Epidemic.* Random House, New York. 1988

Thomson, William (ed). *Medicines from the Earth: A Guide to Healing Plants.* McGraw Hill Book Company. New York. St. Louis. San Francisco. 1978

Wallach, Joel and Boever, Wm. *Diseases of Exotic Animals: Medical and Surgical Management.* W.B. Saunders Publishing Co., Philadelphia. 1983

Wensel, Louise. *Acupuncture for Americans.* Reston Publishing Company, Inc., Reston, Virginia. 1980

Werbach, Melvyn. *Nutritional Influences on Illness: A Sourcebook of Clinical Research.* Third Line Press, Inc., Tarzana, California. 1988

Williams, Lindsey. *You Can Live.* Life and Health Publications, Portland, Oregon. 1989

Spanish Science Terms

algebra	algebra
anatomy	anatomia
anthropology	antropologia
apiculture	apicultura
bacteriology	bacteriologia
biochemistry	bioqu'imica
biology	biologia
botany	bot'anica
chemistry	qu'imica
crystallography	cristalograf'ia
dentistry	dentisteria
embryology	emriologia
entomology	entomolo'gia
geography	geografia
geology	geologia
geometry	geometria
horticulture	horticultura
ichthyology	ictiologia
immunology	inmunologia
insurance	seguros
injection	injecci"on
logic	l'ogica

mathematics	matem'aticas
medicine	medicina
metallurgy	metalurgia
meteorology	meteorologia
mineralogy	mineralogia
neuter	neutro
obstetrics	obstetricia
optics	'optica
ornithology	ornitologia
paleontology	paleontolog'ia
pathology	patologia
pharmacy	farmacia
physics	fisica
physiology	fisiolog'ia
psychoanalysis	psicoan'alisis
psychology	psicolog'ia
psychopathology	psicopatolog'ia
surgery	cirug'ia
veterinary medicine	veterinaria
zoology	zoolog'ia

Other Information

The stress produced by changes in our daily habits have been carefully observed, charted and evaluated by psychologists. It became very obvious that certain changes produced much greater stress than others. A number, according to the severity of the response, was assigned to the thirty-seven most frequent changes in habits.

The stress scale on the following page can be used by you to determine where the personal stresses in your life might lead you. Although it is easily understood when properly examined, many do not recognize that the inability to accommodate stress proceeds possible illness or overwhelming urges. The alcoholic prone will consume more alcohol, the smoker more and the one who finds solace in food will overeat.

Your ability to accommodate stress is directly related to the nutritional balance in your body. This logically explains how one is able to sail through considerable stress without serious consequences while another under similar stress has physical and/or mental breakdowns. It's the chemistry that determines your reactions and you can begin now to enhance your personal chemistry through proper nutrition.

If the stress rating scale shown for you exceeds 150 points of change in 12 months, the chances are one out of two that you might suffer significant illness and a tremendous urge to overeat during the following 24 months. If the amount of change exceeds 300 points in a 12 month period, the chances are better than four out of five that you will suffer significant illness and a tremendous urge to overeat in the succeeding 24 months.

Stress Scale

1.	Death of family member or close friend	100 ______
2.	Divorce	73 ______
3.	Marital separation	65 ______
4.	Personal injury or illness	63 ______
5.	Marriage	53 ______
6.	Fired from job	50 ______
7.	Marital reconciliation	47 ______
8.	Change in health of family member	45 ______
9.	Pregnancy	44 ______
10.	Sex difficulties	40 ______
11.	Gain of a new family member	39 ______
12.	Business adjustment	39 ______
13.	Change in financial state	38 ______
14.	Change in profession or trade	36 ______
15.	Change in number of arguments with spouse	35 ______
16.	Mortgage over $10,000	31 ______
17.	Change in responsibilities at work	30 ______
18.	Son or daughter leaving home	29 ______
19.	Trouble with in-laws	29 ______
20.	Outstanding personal achievement	28 ______
21.	Spouse is laid off work	26 ______
22.	Begin or end school	26 ______
23.	Change in living conditions	25 ______
24.	Revision of personal habits	24 ______
25.	Trouble with boss	23 ______
26.	Change in work hours or conditions	20 ______
27.	Change in residence	20 ______
28.	Change in school	20 ______
29.	Change in recreational activities	19 ______
30.	Change in church activities	19 ______
31.	Change in social activities	18 ______
32.	Mortgage or loan less than $10,000	17 ______
33.	Change in sleeping habits	16 ______
34.	Change in numbers of family get togethers	15 ______
35.	Change in eating habits	15 ______
36.	Vacation	13 ______
37.	Season holidays (Christmas, New Years, etc.)	12 ______

TOTAL ________

Reflexology

The concept of reflexology holds that various organs, nerves, and glands in your body are connected with certain "reflex areas" on the bottoms of your feet, hands and other areas of the body. Moreover, this philosophy claims that by massaging these corresponding areas, prompt relief from a variety of conditions in the body can be obtained. In most instances the thumb, or sometimes a knuckle, is used as the massaging force; although many use vibrators or other external forces.

Considerable credence has been given this work by science, now that we have more or less explained the mechanism by which acupuncture works, since the principle is the same and many physicians are now using acupressure for a variety of conditions, including almost instantaneous relief from headaches and toothaches. This should obviously not be misinterpreted to mean that this methodology will cure the cause of this pain in these two instances, however, in cases of gland or organ congestion, there have been dramatic rehabilitations reported.

The following charts may be of some assistance to you, if you wish to apply some very well authenticated principles of healing your body. There are several techniques such as rotary massage, back and forth massage, probing massage, etc., but the important factor is to find the right spot and it is tender to the touch, massage the area. There is no question that you will find more tender spots on your feet than your hands, but that does not limit the effectiveness of massaging the corresponding area on the hand that you found tender on the foot.

Probably one of the most immediate benefits from reflex massage is the feeling of complete relaxation after the session. Nervous tension, which is so universal in our society, seems to just melt away and you can enjoy deep, restful sleep. These charts may open the door for you to a different way of maintaining health, vitality and the joy of living.

Reflex Chart

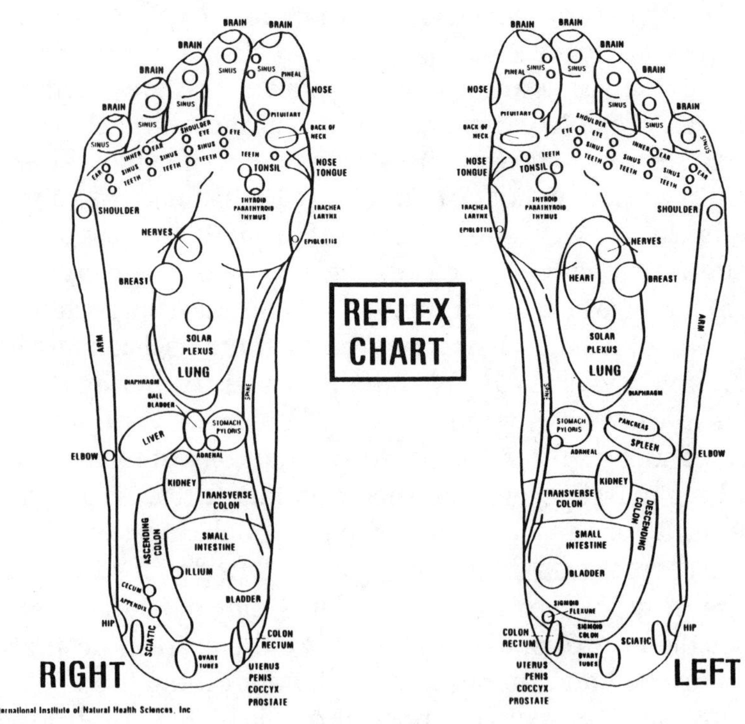

Reflex Chart

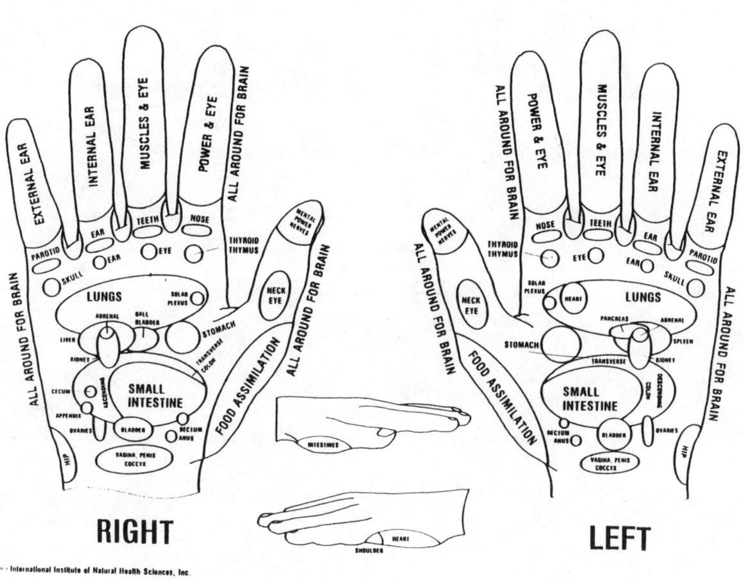

Index

A

abrasions 131
abscess 131
abscence attacks 131
ACE 217, 219, 237, 239, 308
achalasia 131
achloryhydria 132
acne 75, 78, 79, 85, 107
aconite 100, 114, 286
acupuncture 1, 81
adrenal gland exhaust 133
adrenalin 116
A/G ratio 59
AIDS 134
air sick 170
albumin 59
alcoholism 107, 135, 322
allergic shiners 136
allergies 135
allergy test 55
allium cepa 100
alopecia 137
Alzheimer's 263
amblyopia 137
amernorrhea 138
amoebiasis 137
anal abscess 138
anaphylaxsis 138
anemia 139
aneurysm 139
angina 139
anorexia 140
anosmia 141
antibiotics 243
anxiety 141
aphthous stomatitis 141
arnica 148
arsenic toxicity 142
arsenicum album 100
arteriosclerosis 142
aromatherapy 85
athlete's foot 105
asthma 145
arthritis 143
atherosclerosis 145
atopic dermatitis 145
autism 147
autoimmune disorders 147
Avogadro's law 97
ayurvedic medicine 86

B

Bach remedies 88
backache 147
bad breath 148
baldness 148
basophils 55
besores 148

bedwetting 149
bee stings 149
belch, burp and bloat 177
Bell's palsy 150
belladonna 100
benign prostatic hyperplasia 149
biochemics 88
biotin 118
bipolar disorder 151
birth control 86
birth defects 122, 152
bladder infection 192
bladder stones 152
bleeding 153
bleeding bowels 154
bleeding gums 154
bloating 154
blood pressure 12, 17, 20
body odor 155
boils 93, 131, 155
bone pain 155
bone spurs 72
breast cysts 156
brittle nails 156
bronchial asthma 157
bronchitis 157
"brown rice" diet 106
bruises 157
bruxism 158
bryonia 100
BUN 17, 60
BUN/Creatinine ratio 60
burns 158
bursitis 159
butterfly bandage 187, 190

C

calcium 135, 144
calcium/phosphorous ratio 143
calculus 159
calendula 103
cancer 160
candidiasis 165
canker sores 141, 167
car sickness 317
carbuncles 155, 167
carcelim 163
carcinoma 163
cardiac arrythmia 168
cardiomyopathy 168
carpal tunnel syndrome 169
cataracts 170
catarrh 170
CBC 18
CEA 62
ceanothus 103
celiac disease 171
cerebropalsy 172
cerebrovascular disease 172
cervical dysplasia 173
caesarian 120
cesium chloride 162
cestodes 310
chalazion 173
charley horse 274
cheilosis 174
chicken pox 174
chiggers 174

chiropractic 88
chilblains 175
"Chinese restaurant syndrome" 168
chloride 118
choking 280
cholesterol 175
choline 118, 136, 194
chorea 176
chloride 61
chromium 72
chronic fatigue syndrome 165
cirrhosis 258
claudication 143
climacteric 178
cluster headaches 179
CO Q-10 164
cold sore 167, 231
colic 153, 180
colitis 181
colloidal minerals 336
color therapy 88, 93
congested lungs 181
congestive heart failure 182
conjunctivitis 182
constipation 182
contraception 183
convulsions 184
copper 72
cor pulmonare 184
cough 185
cough medicine 116
crabs 185
cradle cap 186
creatinine 60
crohn's disease 186
croup 100, 170
cuts 187
cystic calculi 152
cystic fibrosis 187
cystitis 192

D

dandruff 193
deafness 227
deferential 55
dementia 193
depression 194
dermatitis 195
diabetes 196
diagnosis 67
diaper rash 198
diarrhea 198
dieting 199
diuretic 200
diverticulitis 200
DMSO 164
douche 201
dropsy 182
dysentery 137, 198, 203
dyslexia 203
dysmenorrhea 205
dyspepsia 205, 228, 232, 244

E

ear infection 206
earache 206
EBV 176
ecchymosis 206

eclampsia 292
eczema 145, 195, 207
ejaculation, premature 207
electric shock 209
emesis 210
eosinophils 55
epilepsy 211
epistaxis 277
essential fatty acids 106
exercise equipment 46
exophthalmos 212
eye redness 212

F

failure to thrive 213
farting 213
fatigue 176, 213
fecal sample 13, 64
fertility 214
fever 175, 214
fever blister 167
fibrocystic breast disease 215
fibrocystic disease 156
fingernails 215
fits 184, 211, 216
flatulence 216
flu 175, 216
fluoride 118
flutamide 163
folic acid 73, 118
food allergies 116, 218
fractures 220
freckles 220

G

gall stones 73, 221
gallbladder disease 221
gastric ulcers 316
gelsimium 101
gentiana lutea 102
geographic tongue 222
germanium 162
GGT 62
gingivitis 222, 225, 288
glaucoma 223
globulin 59
glucose 56
glucostick 51
gluten enteropathy 171, 224
goiter 224
goose bump 248
gout 224
grippe 157
growing pains 155, 225
GTT 141
gums, sore 225

H

hair analysis 63
hair loss 225
hangnails 225
hay fever 226
HCT (hematocrit) 21, 54
HDL 57
headaches 73, 179, 226
healing arts 67
hearing loss 227
heart attack 227
heart disease 227

heartburn 228
heating pad 46
hemoglobinometers 52
hemorrhoids 229
hepar sulph 101
hepatitis 229
herbal medicine 95
herpes 231
herpes zoster 231
herpes zoster 174
hiatal hernia 232
hiccoughs 232
hoarseness 233
homeopathy 96
hospitals 327
hoxey herbal formula 163
hydrazine sulfate 162
hydrophobia 294
hydrotherapy 97
hyperacidity 233
hyperactivity 233
hypertension 234
hypoglycemia 235
hypotension 237
hypthyroid 237
hysteria 238

I

iatrogenic 38
icterus 246
immune depression 240
immunization 239
immunotherapy 239
impetigo 240
impotence 241
incontinence 242
indigestion 244
indirect bilirubin 60, 247
infarction 242
infection 243
infertility 243
inflammation 244
infrared light 105
inositol 118
inscription 13
insomnia 245
iodine 73, 173
iron 74
irritable bowel syndrome 245
Isoprinosin 134
itching 246

J

jaundice 246
joint pain 247

K

K (potassium) 61
Kegel's exercise 242, 248
keratomalacia 248
keratosis 248
kernicterus 249
Keshan Disease 76, 125, 168
ketoacidosis 249
kidney disease 249
kidney stones 249
Kilner screen 94
knipping 98
Korsakoff's Syndrome 251

kwashiorkor 251

L

labor 252, 292
laceration 187
lactase deficiency 252
lactation 252
lactobacillus 167
laetrile 162
laryngitis 233, 253
laxative 200, 253
laying-on-of-hands 94
LD 260
LDH 22
LDL 58
lead poisoning 254
learning disorder 203, 254
Legionnaires' disease 254
lentigo-maligna melanoma 255
leptospirosis 255
leukemia 256
leukorrhea 256
lice 257
life expectancy 257
light therapy 93
liver disease 258
liver spots 133
lockjaw 259
lups 259
lyme arthritis 260
lyme disease 260
lymphoma 261

M

macrobiotics 105
magnesium 144
malabsorption 171
malignancy 261
malnutrition 261
manganese 74, 118
manipulation 92
mania 262
materia medica 100
MCH 22, 54
MCHC 54
MCV 54
measles 262
megavitamin therapy 106
melancholia 238
melanoma 255
melasma 263
memory loss 193, 263
menarche 264
meningitis 265
meningocele 265
Menke's kinky hair syndrome 266
menopause 266
mercury poisoning 266
metabolic therapy 267
methadone 267
microscope 45, 137
migraine headaches 268
miscarriage 268
mitral valve prolapse 269
molybdenum 118
Monckeberg's arteriosclerosis 269

mongolism 269
monocytes 55
morning sickness 270
mosquitoes 270
mother tincture 100
mucoviscidosis 187
multiple sclerosis 271
mumps 272
muscle cramps 274
muscular dystrophy 273

N

nasal catarrh 179, 275
nat mur 103
nat sulph 103
naturopathy 107
nausea 275
N.D. 107
negative ion 108
neoplasm 160
nervous heart 275
nervous tension 276
neuralgia 276
neutrophil 55
niacin 151, 176
nightblindness 276
night terrors 277
nightmares 277
nitric acid 102
noblemen 2
nontropical sprue 23
nosebleed 277
numbness 278
nutritional secondary
hyperparathyroidism 283
nux vomica 241

O

OB/GYN 119
obesity 278
oligospermia 281
omphalocele 281
ophthalmoscope 170
organic brain syndrome 282
ornithosis 283
osteitis fibrosa 283
osteoarthritis 283
osteopathy 109
osteoporosis 284
otitis 285
otoscope 44
oxygen 116

P

PABA 75
pain 285
pain killers 114
palpitations 286
panic attacks 141
parasites 286
parkinsonism 287
parrot fever 283
PDR 14
peptic ulcer 288
periodontal disease 288
pharmacy 113
phlebitis 289
phosphorus 75, 118
pica 289
piles 290

pilonidal cyst 290
pimples 290
pink eye 212
placenta previa 119, 122
plumbism 254
PMS 156, 195, 290
poison ivy 291
polycrests 100
polyerga 164
potassium 75, 118
potencies 96
poor circulation 291
post partum hemorrhage 291
pox 291
pregnancy labor 292
pregnancy toxemia 292
premenstrual syndrome 290
prostate hyperplasia 292
pruritis 246
psoriasis 293
public health 333, 336
pulsatilla 100, 213, 214
pyorrhea 293
pyridoxine 76, 118

Q

Q fever 293
quinsy 294

R

rabbit fever 294
rabies 294
rainbow healing 94
rachitic rosary 295
radial nerve palsy 295
rape 296
Raynaud's disease 297
RBC 25, 246
receding gums 154
rectal itching 297
referrals 323
reflex hammer 43, 169
reflexology 85, 109
reflux 228, 232
regional enteritis 186
repertory 100
Reye's syndrome 298
rheumatic fever 298
rheumatism 298
rheumatoid arthritis 298
rhus tox 104
ribavirin 134
riboflavin 118
rickets 300
ringworm 300
rocky mountain
spotted fever 301
rolfing 109
roseola 302
rubber gloves 84

S

sarcoma 160
scabies 302
scarlatina 302
scarlet fever 302
schizophrenia 303
sciatica 303
scoliosis 303
Schuessler cell salts 88

scurvy 304
sea sickness 170
sebaceous cyst 304
seborrheic dermatitis 304
seizures 184
semmelwise 121
senila dementia 305
SGOT 26, 230
shark skin 305
shingles 305
skin ailments 306
SLE 259
smelling salts 116
sodium 23
solar-chrome salt bags 94
sore throat 306
sphygmomanometer 43
spider bite 307
spina bifida 265
sprain 306
sties 212
strains 307
stress 307
stroke 308
subscription 13
supplement program 118
sweat test 308
sweat test table 189
swimmer's ear 308
syphillis 309
syringe 45
syrup of ipecac 116

T

tachycardia 309
tapeworms 310
tardrive dyskinesia 310
tartar 159
teeth discoloration 311
teething 311
terentula 102
testicular atrophy 311
thallium poisoning 312
thermometer 42
thiamine 118
thrush 312
thumb forceps 44
tick fever 301
tinnitus 313
TMJ 311
tonsilitis 314
toothache 314
torticollis spasmodic 314
toxemia 292
toxic shock syndrome 314
toxoplasmosis 315
triglycerides 316
TSS 314

U

ulcer 316
ulcerative colitis 317
ultraviolet 45, 105
umbilical hernia 281
urine tests 68
urine therapy 110
urticaria 317

V

vaginitis 317
valeriana 103
Van Leeuwenhoek 4
varicose veins 289, 317
vertigo 317
vitamin A 78, 118
vitamin B-1 77, 118
vitamin B-12 77, 118
vitamin C 78, 118
vitamin D 78, 118
vitamin E 78, 118
vitamin K 79, 118
vitamins & minerals 118
vitiligo 318
vomiting 210

W

Wallach' s vertigo 318
warts 318
WBC 27
weight 27
weight loss 318
wen 304
white spots, fingernails 318
whooping cough 170
worms 319
wounds 319
wryneck 314

X

xerophthalmia 248
xylocaine 114

Y

yang 82
yellow fever 5, 271
yin 82
yoga 110

Z

zits 319
zinc 79, 118
zumba 209

Special Savings Offers!

Save on BOOKS

Let's Play Doctor

The Book That "Orthodox" Doctors Couldn't Kill "How To" maximize your genetic potential for health and longevity.

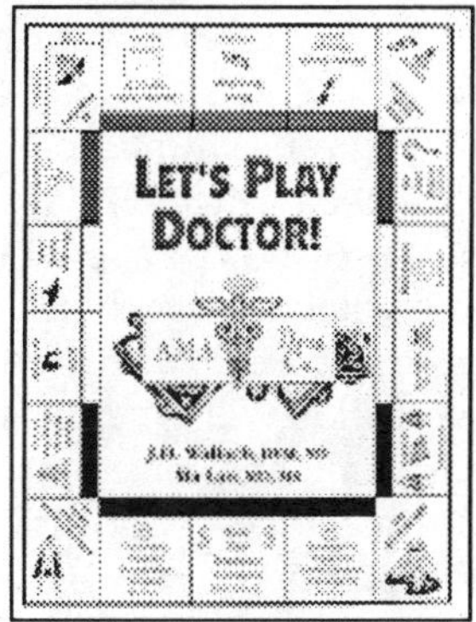

- Become your own primary health care provider
- Learn the Alternative Healing Arts
- Establish your own health clinic
- Establish a home pharmacy
- Home Surgery

■ LET'S PLAY DOCTOR (Book) **$12.95**

10 or more **$7.00** each

Rare Earths Forbidden Cures

Their Secrets of Health and Longevity

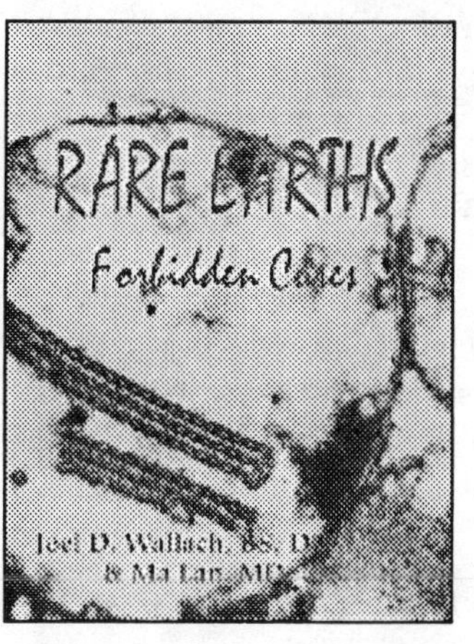

The definitive home reference on minerals, mineral deficiencies and their relationship to:

- Degenerative Diseases
- Learning Disabilities
- Criminal Behavior
- Hyperactivity
- Birth Defects
- Addiction
- Food Binges
- Depression
- Infertility and more!

■ RARE EARTHS: Forbidden Cures **$19.95**

10 or more **$12.00** each

Special Savings Offers!

Save on AUDIO ALBUMS

Let's Play Doctor (The Workshop)

To help you reach your maximum genetic potenial for health and longevity, Dr. Joel Wallach and Dr. Ma Lan have put together a 220 minute workshop which tells you "how to avoid the land mines" and what positive things you can do for yourself and your loved ones. This workshop will save you from unnecessary pain and misery and an untimely death and as a bonus it will save you a lot of money!

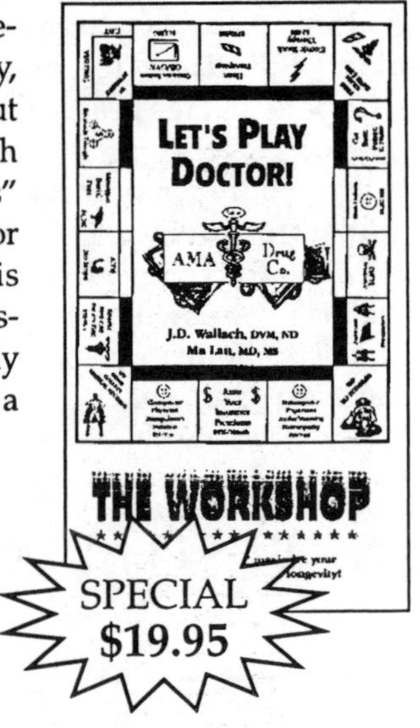

- LET'S PLAY DOCTOR WORKSHOP
  (3 Audio Cassettes) ~~$24.95~~
  10 or more **$12.95**

Air Strike (Audio)

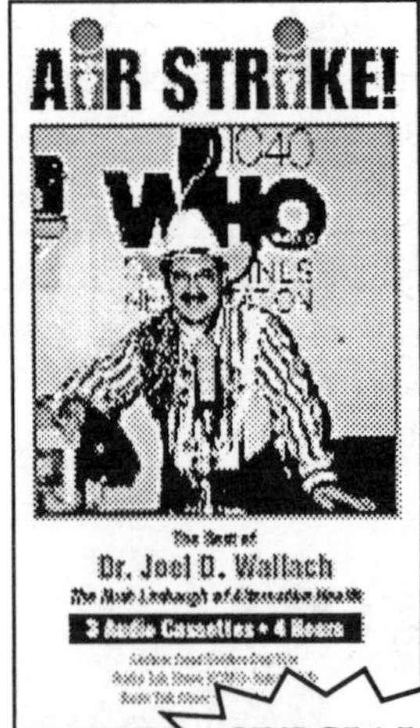

Dr. Joel D. Wallach, the Rush Limbaugh of alternative health delivers an information "Air Strike" right on target using doctors' obituaries, medical and nutritional facts and two top regional radio talk shows. Rush would be proud!

The Best of Dr. Joel D. Wallach, The Rush Limbaugh of Alternative health on 3 Audio Cassettes, over 4 hours of lectures - Dead Doctors Don't Lie. Talk radio KCMO - Kansas City, and WHO - De Moines.

- AIR STRIKE (3 Audio Cassettes)
  ~~$24.95~~
  10 or more **$12.95**

Dead Athletes Don't Lie

(3 Audio Cassettes)

"Dr. Joel Wallach delivers a 1-2-3 punch in this latest audio series! A must have for any serious athlete who wants to know the secrets to sports longevity."

Mike "Stinger" Glenn
Point Guard - Atlanta Hawks (1982-1985)

Dr. Joel D. Wallach, delivers an educational as well as a motivational presentation concerning proper nutrition and sports performance. Using athlete obituaries, medical and nutritional facts and interviews with sports greats Mike "Stinger" Glenn and Dr. Don "Fist of Thunder" Nielsen, listeners will discover the secrets to sports health, longevity and greatness.

- DEAD ATHLETES DON'T LIE
(3 Audio Cassettes)
~~$24.95~~

SPECIAL
$19.95

10 or more **$12.95**

More Audio Cassettes!

- Dead Doctors Don't Lie I (Audio)
1 to 10 **$2.50** each • 10 or more **$1.75** each
- Dead Doctors Don't Lie II (Audio)
1 to 10 **$2.50** each • 10 or more **$1.75** each
- Trust Me I'm A Doctor (Audio)
1 to 10 **$3.00** each • 10 or more **$2.00** each

Save on VIDEOS & Magazine

Dead Doctors Don't Lie

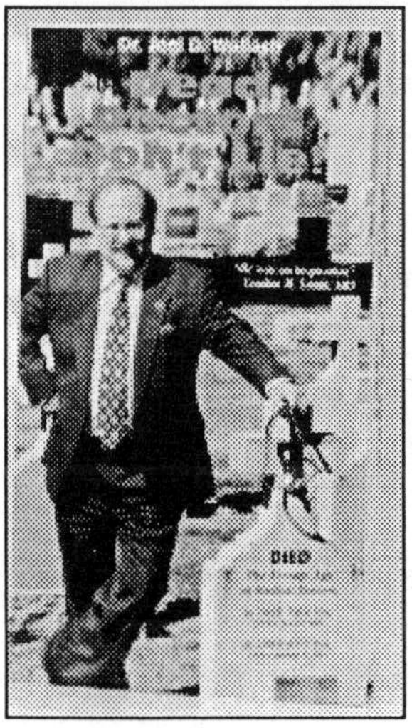

This one is a must for your video library, a classic 2-hour lecture by Dr. Wallach on why you should and can take charge of your own health! Dr. Wallach uses physicians' obituaries to prove his point.

■ DEAD DOCTORS DON'T LIE Video Lecture (1995 Revision)
$24.95

10 or more **$15.95**

NEW!

Trust Me, I'm A Doctor

Dr. Wallach will show you that you have the genetic potential to live beyond the age of 100. But, the average American will fall short by 24 years and the average American doctor only lives to the age of 68. For some reason however, we have been brainwashed to trust our doctor blindly and not to question their advice. Learn about the importance of minerals and how they are beneficial to your health. See how the only way to guarantee that you are getting enough is by taking vitamins and mineral supplements.

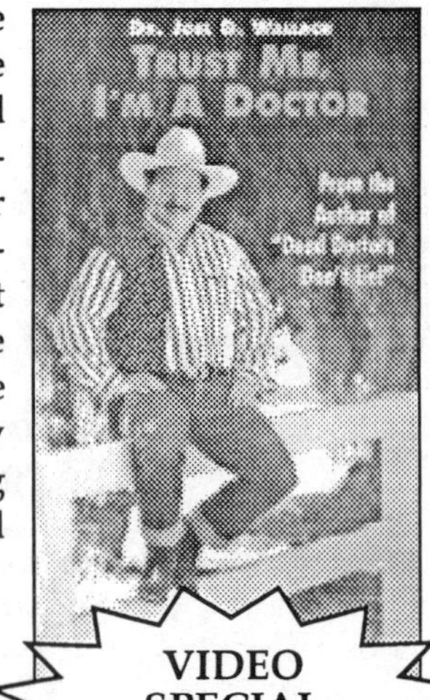

■ TRUST ME I'M A DOCTOR
(1997 version)

10 or more **$15.95**

VIDEO SPECIAL **$24.95**

Health Consciousness Magazine

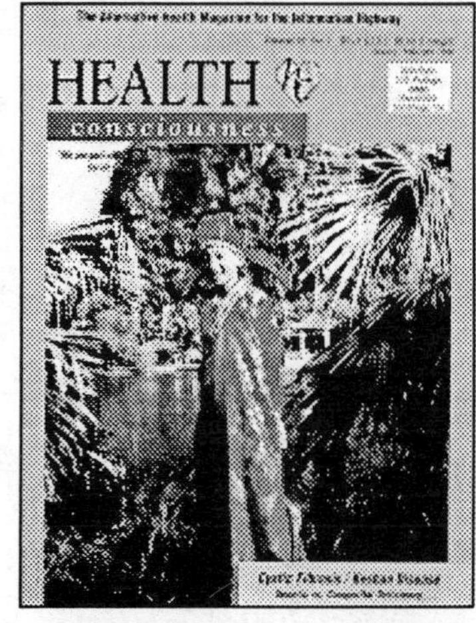

THE ALTERNATIVE HEALTH MAGAZINE FOR THE INFORMATION SUPERHIGHWAY

Raise awareness, understanding and knowledge... Health news for both the lay and professional reader... International viewpoints in pioneers in Alternative Medicine... Exploring the physical, mental, emotional and spiritual frontiers of medicine... Featuring Health News updates...

Health Consciousness is published bi-monthly. Subscription rate is **$18**/year (six issues). Outside U.S. **$32**/year by surface mail, **$80** by air. Sample introductory copy will be sent upon request and upon receipt of **$3** (**$6** foreign) for postage and handling.

Let's Play Doctor Computer Database

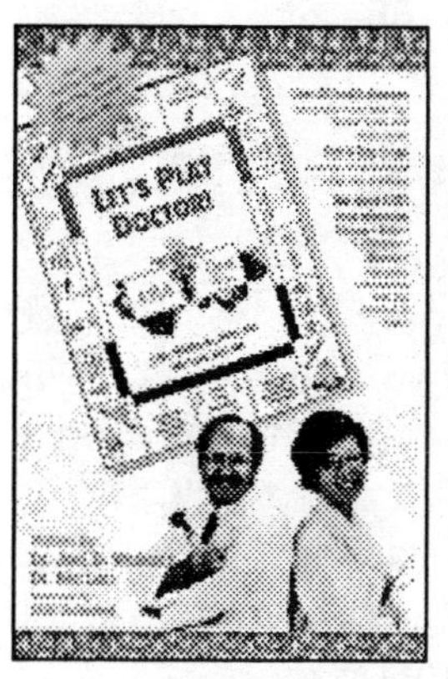

Gain the upperhand on your health the easy way with Dr. Wallach's Let's Play Doctor - Computer Database. Over 400 health disorders! Fast and easy to use. A simple to understand computer database... Has over 7, 800 cross references... Vitamins... Herbs... O_2 Therapies... Minerals... Complete information with the touch of a finger! Written by Dr. Joel D. Wallach and Dr. Ma Lan. Database by IAM Unlimited.

HARDWARE REQUIREMENTS

Macintosh® 68020 or greater, System 7 or later, 4MB RAM, 8MB Recommended, 3MB Hard Disk space available, System 7.1.2 or later PowerMac. IBM®/Compatibles - Microsoft® Windows 3.0 or greater, 2MB RAM Minimum, 3MB Hard Disk space available.

■ LET'S PLAY DOCTOR (Computer Database) **$59.95**

Dr. Wallach's "Pig Arthritis" Formula

- 5 oz. calcium enriched Orange juice
- 1 oz. plant-derived colloidal minerals
- 1 oz. vitamin / amino acid / colloidal mineral mix
- Take 7 oz. twice daily at breakfast and dinner time with $^1/_2$ oz. or 4-6 Willamette Valley Gelatin Cap®

7 1/2 oz. TOTAL MIX

To get all 90 nutrients, add Willamette Valley Liquid Calcium Caps® and Willamette Valley Flax Oil Caps®

You must try this formula if you have arthritis or osteoporosis!

This recipe is brought to you by Dr. Joel Wallach
To inquire or order books, tapes, videos or Virgin Earth™ products, please call 1-800-755-4656.

Become your own primary health care provider!

The ultimate test of a product is that the people who sell it use it themselves — like the financial advisor who invests his own money in the same funds that he recommends to his clients. Young people and old, including Dr. Wallach himself, fuel up daily with liquid, colloidal vitamins and minerals. And for the price of a pop and a bagel each day, you, too, can give your body the 90 essential nutrients. Call for more information!

Judy DeVilbiss
350 Maher Road
Watsonville CA 95076
888-352-7500/831-728-3500

E-mail: w ... ach.com

Order Form

Phone Orders
1-800-755-4656

Date	Phone	Fax / E-Mail

Last Name	First Name	Middle Initial
Street Address		Apt. No.
City		
State		Zip Code

Qty.	Description	Price	Total	
		Sub-Total		
		Shipping & Handling (See chart)		
		5% Processing Fee		
		TOTAL		

Method of Payment

- ☐ MasterCard
- ☐ American Express
- ☐ Discover
- ☐ Check
- ☐ Visa
- ☐ Money Order

Shipping & Handling

FOR ORDERS TOTALLING	ADD
Up to $25.00	$5.00
$25.01 - $50.00	$6.00
$50.01 - $100.00	$8.00
$101.00 - $200.00	$10.00
$201.00 - $500.00	$14.00
Over $500.00	Please call for rates

Account Number

Exp. Date

Cardmember Name *(Please Print)*

Signature

X